More Advanced Praise for
Out of Darkness

Postpartum psychosis is a co. plex and serious illness that is fortunately gaining more attention by researchers, practitioners and families alike. Jennifer Moyer's deeply personal testimony is helpful in that it offers both a window and a mirror to the disease. Like Scott Stossel's recent book, *My Age of Anxiety*, Moyer provides amazing insight as to what it is like to experience the disabling aspects of severe postpartum illness. Her words also offer a reflection for care providers, psychiatrists, family members, and others, that hopefully will lead to more informed care. Moyer takes us on a tumultuous journey, one that she survived...giving hope for all.

Laurence Kruckman, PhD, Professor Emeritus, Anthropology

Jennifer Moyer's book provides a much needed addition to the body of literature about postpartum psychosis. Whereas my book includes several brief first-person "snapshots" of this illness, Moyer's provides an in-depth look, including the ongoing process of recovery and the consequences of having had this illness. I applaud Moyer's bravery and her generosity in being willing to share her story to help others."

Teresa M. Twomey, author Understanding Postpartum Psychosis: A Temporary Madness

Jennifer Hentz Moyer's *A Mother's Climb out of Darkness: A Story About Overcoming Postpartum Psychosis* is a rare and powerful in-depth look into the world of postpartum psychosis and the on-going process of maternal mental health. We are fully invited in on this sometime harrowing journey that provides hope to those who may feel broken. This book is also an important must read for those who work with children, families and within the mental health field. Throughout her climb, Ms. Moyer shares from her unique perspective insight with windows of opportunity to improve helping to build healthy families right from the start.

> Sonia Murdock, Executive Director and Co Founder Postpartum Resource Center of New York, Inc.

With grace and courage, Jennifer Moyer eloquently invites us into the world of postpartum psychosis, a world of anguish where there often are no words. But hers is a story, not of tragedy, but one of hope and promise as she skillfully weaves personal narrative together with the real facts about perinatal psychiatric illness. "A Mother's Climb out of Darkness" will help increase your understanding about the most misunderstood of postpartum disorders.

> Diana Lynn Barnes, Psy.D , editor, *Women's Reproductive Mental Health Across the Lifespan* (Springer, 2014).

Jennifer's story provides hope to any woman and her partner who experiences postpartum psychosis. She is honest about her struggles, and doesn't promise a quick fix. No matter how dark your despair, this book shows that if you are patient, and take small steps, a brighter dawn is ahead.

Graeme Cowan, Resilience and Mental Health Speaker and Author of Back From The Brink

Jennifer Moyer has written a powerful, poignant, and often painful memoir. Her journey through postpartum psychosis and beyond is an important and historic addition to the mental health literature. Jennifer has documented her struggles with honesty, insight, and love.

Jane Honikman, MS, Founder, Postpartum Support International

"What an important and relevant document this is! The first step to medical and/or legal assistance for those who suffer from postpartum issues is to get the message out. Jennifer Moyer does just that! Congratulations."

George J. Parnham, Attorney to Andrea Yates

As a mental health advocate, I know the best way to foster acceptance of mental health challenges is to hear the struggle and the triumph of overcoming them from those that have experienced it first-hand. Jennifer bravely shares her story to bring compassion and understanding to an experience that many have shied away from identifying with because of fear and/or shame. Her story serves as a reminder that despite the diagnosis, the prognosis, and the internal and societal conflicts ahead, individuals living with mental health challenges, can and do get better.

Dana Foglesong, Peer Recovery Solutions

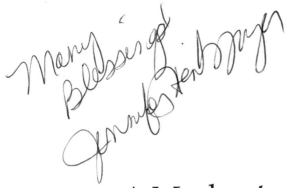

A Mother's Climb out of Darkness

A Story about Overcoming Postpartum Psychosis

Jennifer Hentz Moyer

Foreword by

Samantha Meltzer-Brody, MD

Associate Professor and Director of the Perinatal Psychiatry Program, UNC Center for Women's Mood Disorders

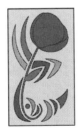

Praeclarus Press, LLC

©2014 Jennifer Hentz Moyer. All rights reserved.

www.PraeclarusPress.com

Praeclarus Press, LLC
2504 Sweetgum Lane
Amarillo, Texas 79124 USA
806-367-9950
www.PraeclarusPress.com

All rights reserved. No part of this publication may be reproduced or transmitted in any form, or by any means, electronic or mechanical, including photocopy, recording, stored in a database, or any information storage, or put into a computer, without the prior written permission from the publisher.

DISCLAIMER

The information contained in this publication is advisory only and is not intended to replace sound clinical judgment or individualized patient care. The author disclaims all warranties, whether expressed or implied, including any warranty as the quality, accuracy, safety, or suitability of this information for any particular purpose.

ISBN: 9781939807144

©2014. Jennifer Hentz Moyer. All rights reserved.

Cover Design: Ken Tackett
Acquisition & Development: Kathleen Kendall-Tackett
Copy Editing: Nancy Tamms
Layout & Design: Todd Rollison
Operations: Scott Sherwood

My thanks to God, my family, and all of my friends for never giving up on me, even in the darkest moments

This book is dedicated to my mother, my husband, my son, and all the women and families who have been struck by postpartum psychosis.

Mental illness related to the birth process is a prevalent and greatly misunderstood medical and psychological disorder among childbearing women. The impact it can have on a woman and her family is profound and painful, wreaking havoc on the lives of all those it touches.

If undiagnosed and left untreated, it can lead to tragedies, such as chronic affective disorders, inadequate infant-mother bonding, marital discord, divorce, suicide, infanticide, child neglect and abuse, and substance abuse.

-Jane Honikman, MS, Founder, Postpartum Support International

A percentage of the proceeds from the sale of this book will be donated to non-profit organizations that are working toward raising public awareness, providing education, and supporting the prevention and treatment of mental illness related to childbearing, and mental illness, in general.

Forever With Me

Kate Gaffney

Dedicated to Catherine M. Hentz

You came by to see me just yesterday
You had something to tell me but you just couldn't say
So you showed me a picture of when we met last time
When you told me that you knew I was doing just fine
And I expressed my love with a kiss and embrace
Unaware that I'd never again see your face

My mother she called me quite early today
I cried when she told me you'd just gone away
But a feeling of ease it ran straight through my blood
When I knew where you were at home with your Lord
And after times of heartache and surfacing strong
You've found your way back to where you belong

We share a name and a bond for all time
And I know that you'll always be right by my side
And when the nights grow dark, bitter, and cold
I'll feel you near me I won't be alone
There's no more reason for living in fear
Your faith has shown me how to take it from here

©2005 Kate Gaffney. Printed with permission.

Table of Contents

Foreword

Jennifer Moyer poignantly and bravely describes her battle with postpartum psychosis and the difficulties she encountered finding compassionate and knowledgeable care for this devastating disorder. Postpartum psychosis has a prevalence of 0.1% in the general population, and is often the first manifestation of bipolar disorder in women. In those women with a known history of bipolar disorder (prior to pregnancy), the risk of postpartum psychosis is significantly greater. In Jennifer's case, postpartum psychosis was the first episode of her bipolar illness. She struggled with symptoms of bipolar illness for several years. Today, she manages her illness well. As I write this, with proper care and treatment, she has been stable for more than six years and functions at a high level.

In her book, *A Mother's Climb Out of Darkness*, Jennifer recounts the onset of her postpartum psychosis, and the pain she and her family endured. She is able to give an honest, and at times, deeply disturbing view of her mind during episodes of psychosis including her paranoia and delusions. This stark account of her suffering gives a voice to the women and their families who have suffered with this horrible illness.

Unfortunately, until rather recently, there has been both a lack of awareness and insufficient mental health services available to women with mental illness during pregnancy and the postpartum period. This has led to enormous suffering and inappropriate treatment resulting in poor outcomes and needless suffering. Thankfully, the tide is turning and knowledge about women's reproductive mood disorders is increasing. Many academic medical centers now have specific programs in women's mental health and reproductive mood disorders, and national advocacy organizations, such as Postpartum Support International (PSI), provide education and support on a wide scale level.

Thankfully, over the past few years, the United States has seen some significant positive changes that will help increase awareness and support of women with perinatal mental illness. For example, the 2010 passage of the Melanie Blocker Stokes Safe Mothers Act, as part of the Health Insurance Reform Act, passed Congress in March 2010, and established a federal commitment to combating postpartum depression through new research, education initiatives, and voluntary support services programs. This landmark bill has led to important new initiatives and innovative programs, and has given hope to many women and their families.

At the University of North Carolina at Chapel Hill, our Perinatal Psychiatry Program has created a comprehensive program to include specialized outpatient, inpatient, and research programs for women with perinatal psychiatric illness. Our Perinatal Psychiatry Inpatient Unit (PPIU) is the first in the United States and opened in August 2011. It should be noted that the opening of the PPIU at UNC comes only 50 years after the first mother-baby psychiatry unit was opened in Europe (Great Britain). Thus, the United States is now making slow but steady progress toward providing women with specialized perinatal psychiatry treatment services that are critically important for the health of the women, children, and families.

I believe that Jennifer Moyer's book will provide those that suffer with severe postpartum mental illness with hope and inspiration, and ultimately, it will help increase awareness about the devastating impact of untreated or inadequately treated mental illness. There is so much more work that needs to be done, but Jennifer's book is an important step in the right direction.

Samantha Meltzer-Brody, MD, MPH
Chapel Hill, North Carolina
February 4, 2013

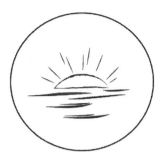

Acknowledgments

First and foremost, I must thank my husband and all of the members of my family. Through the years they have given me love and support without which I would not be the woman I am today. I am forever grateful to them as well as to all of those who have provided me with support, encouragement, and hope. They are too numerous to mention individually.

A special thank you to my son, without the inspiration and purpose he gave me to make it through this journey, I would have no story to share. He is amazing and has grown into an awesome young man.

The years involved in bringing this book to publication are numerous. Over these years in the process of trying to get the book published, I received so many rejections that I lost count. There were times that I would put the process aside only for something or someone to bring it to the surface again. But one day I got to the point that I threw my hands up in the air in frustration, calling out that either the desire in me to publish this book be taken from me or somehow make it happen. I gave it one more shot and clearly, God heard my plea because not long after that day back in 2011, I was led to Maryann Karinch with the Rudy Agency.

Maryann was the first person in the publishing business that saw the power of this story clear enough that she offered the direction and guidance I needed to enable me to move forward with this project. If it was not for her dedication and passion, I would have never moved forward. I am eternally grateful for her. Through Maryann I was led to another individual, Judith Bailey. Without Judith's expertise in editing and her commitment to have this book come to life and be published, the project probably never would have proceeded in the right direction. She is a kindred spirit and my appreciation to her is beyond words. My thanks also goes out to my dear friend, Kathryne Waller, whose freelance writing skills helped me fine tune the end result that you now hold in your hands.

My goal in writing this book is that it brings better understanding of not only mental illness related to childbearing, but mental illness in general.

This goal would have no chance at being achieved without having a conversation with Wendy Davis back in October 2013. As a result, I learned of Kathleen Kendall-Tackett with Praeclarus Press. Kathleen's passion for women's health issues is the driving force in this book being published.

My desire is that this book brings encouragement to those who have been touched by mental health challenges related to childbearing. I also wish for it to increase the awareness, prevention, and proper treatment of mental illness, stomping out stigma along the way. I have discovered many things during my journey with mental illness, so I believe that no matter where the reader is on his or her journey, this book will bring them hope and inspiration along the way.

I share my story so others can learn that it is possible to overcome darkness.

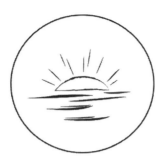

Chapter One

Descent into Darkness

In front of my neighbors, many of whom had come out of their houses to see what was happening, several strong men wrestled me to the ground, strapped me onto a gurney, and loaded me into a waiting ambulance. I cried out for help, but no one responded. All I could do was move my head, and it was hard to see through my confusion and the pulsing colored lights. But off to the side I thought I saw my husband talking to several people. It looked like him, but Michael wouldn't just let this happen to me, would he? Were my college friend and my doctor in the crowd milling about on the lawn? I remember calling out, pleading for assistance, but no one responded. Where was my 2-month-old son? I had tried to protect him as I was assaulted, but now I couldn't see him anywhere. What had they done with him? Why was this happening?

The doors closed, cutting off my view, and we sped away into the night. The two men in the ambulance with me laughed at my fear and confusion. "Maybe the carbon monoxide exhaust will help knock her out," said one as he settled into position at my feet. I knew I was beyond all earthly aid, with only my faith to uphold me. "*All things are possible through Christ who strengthens me.*" I chanted the verse over and over to myself. It was a prayer for strength and the only thing I had left.

After a time, the ambulance came to a stop. Restrained as I was, I could make out little of my surroundings, and what I could see was completely unfamiliar. But it looked like we'd arrived at a hospital and that gave me a desperate idea. If my abductors were going to pretend to be real medical personnel, maybe I could use this. I demanded to be taken to the hospital at which I'd been employed. People would know me there. I would be safe.

No one responded or even acknowledged that I'd spoken.

They wheeled my gurney into the hospital entrance and left me alone in a corridor for hours. The only movement I could make was to turn my head from side to side. This did not allow me to see much. Hurried people, dressed as medical personnel, would occasionally pass by me and I could see others farther down the hall, but no one would respond to my questions or requests for information. It was as if I was mute and invisible. Slowly, I began to suspect that I would die right there and that no one I loved would ever know what had happened to me. Worst of all, I knew I had failed my beautiful, innocent baby boy. Protecting him had been my job. With the tears streaming down my face, I continued my chant softly. *"I can do all things through Christ who strengthens me. I can do all things through Christ who strengthens me."*

Suddenly, I heard a familiar voice and felt a gentle touch. My friend Dianne appeared, as if out of nowhere. Then I remembered. She'd been at my house earlier in the evening, before everything started. She was my friend from college and I hadn't seen her in years. But she'd come to see us that night. At least I thought she had. I couldn't remember why now and I was glad to see her, but it all seemed so strange. Until she spoke I thought I might be dreaming.

"I saw someone I know who works here," she said. "I asked him to keep an eye out for you."

I knew she meant to be kind and was grateful to her, but her words brought me no comfort. I was desperate to know what was happening to my baby, and assurances that he was okay seemed meaningless. I was his protection. How could he be safe if I was not with him? Where was he? And where was my husband?

I would find out much later that the police officers and paramedics had directed Michael to take our son to the emergency room for drug testing. Despite Michael and Dianne's assurances otherwise, the paramedics had concluded I was most likely under the influence of an illicit drug that might harm my son. Drug-induced psychosis was something they saw all too often and they had no other explanation for my behavior.

Michael thought the idea was ridiculous, but he complied.

The next thing I remember is being attacked. I was lying on a bed in a small room and two men were holding me down. A third person, a woman, was trying to inject a needle into my arm. Fearing poison, I struggled against them. "Wow, she's strong," I heard one of them say, but it didn't matter. They won and I felt the needle slide into my arm. "Why are you doing this?" I asked. "What have I done wrong?"

No one answered. No one explained. No one said anything at all. Since I wasn't wearing either my contacts or glasses, their faces were blurred. They strapped my arms to the bed and left me alone. I was too exhausted even to chant and the darkness closed in around me.

I don't know how much time passed before I awoke. It was dark and my vision was blurry, but I could make out a woman sitting in a chair by the doorway. My mouth and throat were parched, but I managed to call out to her. "Please, help me," I pleaded. "Please call my father."

No answer. I tried again. Finally, the woman said, "You are okay." That was all she would say. I continued to plead with her for help, for information about my son, but received only silence in return. My mind raced. It was clear I was being watched, but I had no idea why. What did they want from me? What had they done with my baby?

The next thing I remember is sitting with a man in a larger room. There are other chairs in the room and people I do not know are sitting in them. No one says anything but the man. He tells me that he is with me because I am under a 24-hour suicide watch. Suicide watch? The idea strikes me as absurd. I am not suicidal; I've been fighting for my life and my son's life. The man tells me that I need to let the doctor know I don't want to harm myself.

"What doctor?" I ask. I haven't seen a doctor. The man tells me her name and that she is pregnant with her fourth child. That makes me feel a little better, but I'm not sure this isn't a dream.

It wasn't. I got to meet the doctor later that day. She came into my room with another woman, whom she did not introduce and who said nothing at all. They both sat on my bed.

The doctor seemed nice enough on the surface, but I could tell she was uncomfortable around me. She kept looking at me suspiciously, as if she expected me to do something odd or scary. "How strange," I said to myself. "I'm the one with reason for distrust, but she seems afraid."

Carefully, as if she was talking to a small child, the doctor explained that some women experience depression after having a baby. She began to ask me a series of questions.

Most I no longer recall, but finally she came to, "Do you want to hurt yourself or your baby?"

I thought she was crazy. I wasn't depressed and I had been fighting to save my baby. Didn't she understand that? What would she have done if a bunch of strange men had shown up at her house, taken her child out of her arms, and forcibly abducted her? Then it dawned on me: This woman was not to be trusted. She was part of whatever was happening to me. I listened without comment as she told me that I would have to take a few tests. She didn't tell me why or explain what the tests were supposed to reveal, and I didn't ask. I was pretty sure by then that I wouldn't get an answer anyway.

I was in a psychiatric hospital. That much the doctor would say. She said that my husband and baby were okay. I didn't trust this information and it didn't answer the questions swirling in my head. I had done nothing wrong. Why was I being treated as a prisoner? What did they want from me? I had to get out of that place and back to my baby. I made up my mind to be as cooperative as possible.

They gave me two pills each day. No one told me why the pills had been prescribed or what would happen if I swallowed them. I could think of only one reason they would hide this from me. Obviously, the pills would harm or even kill me. Perhaps they were meant to make me passive or unable to remember what had been done to me. But it was important that the doctor and hospital staff did not know I was aware of what they were up to, so I pretended to take the medication. Then, I would walk back to my room, remove the pills from my mouth, and flush them down the toilet.

Looking back now, I can see how much of my fear might have been alleviated if the people who treated me had explained what was happening. Even today, I'm not sure why they didn't. Perhaps they thought I was unable to understand. But I can tell you for sure that explanations would have helped. Being treated with dignity and respect would have helped. Medication alone was not enough. As it was, the lack of information only fed my fears and increased my determination to escape.

Still, the familiar hospital routine was reassuring in itself. It was something I was used to and that helped calm the worst of my fears. Of course, I was distrustful of everyone around me, but I was determined to hide it. A familiar environment made this much easier. It must have appeared to the doctor and hospital staff that I was responding well to the medication. My family seemed relieved. No one had any idea that I had actually taken none of the pills. I would do anything I had to do to escape my prison and find my baby. My spiritual strength supported me and gave me courage.

I continued pumping my breast milk in the hospital because I planned to continue breastfeeding when I got home. Before the doctor would agree to discharge me, though, I had to take the series of tests she had told me about. The first was a questionnaire. There were a lot of questions and I had a hard time concentrating, but I managed to weigh my answers and come up with responses I thought would satisfy them.

The second test of the series was harder. The woman administering the test asked me to look at pictures on flash cards and tell her what I saw. Since the pictures were simply differently shaped inkblots, I had no idea what they wanted me to say. What answers would be "right" and get me out of the hospital? I struggled to come up with answers that sounded "normal."

I must have done well enough since the hospital staff pronounced me stable and discharged me after four nights in the hospital. They told me that I no longer had to take medication and could resume breastfeeding my baby. I hid a little grim amusement since I'd been flushing the medication.

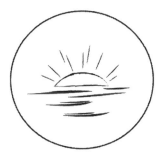

Chapter 2

Fear Becomes Reality

I was so glad to be home and to be reunited with my family. I started breastfeeding again and my son seemed healthy and content. My worry that our separation had harmed him began to fade. All went well for about a week, until I began having trouble sleeping. My mind seemed to stay in constant disorder and the fears began to return. This time, though, I was not just afraid that I would die and someone would take my son. I was also haunted by terrible memories of being attacked and imprisoned. I did not understand what was happening to my mind and why I had been taken to the hospital. It was as if some evil presence had attacked me and would strike again if I showed any sign of weakness. I tried desperately to hold things together.

One evening, about two weeks after I came home from the hospital, I asked Michael, "Do you remember that television show, *The Twilight Zone*?"

"Yes," he replied.

"Well, that's how I feel," I said. "I feel as if I'm living in another dimension."

I think he thought I was joking. I couldn't blame him. I felt as though I'd been dropped into an alien world where things only looked familiar. How could I help him understand what was happening to me when I didn't? I said no more.

Michael and I were trying to make our family life as normal as possible, so we accepted an invitation to my niece's piano recital. It would also give us the opportunity to see several members of my family who lived about an hour away. I needed to feel some control in my life, so I insisted on driving, but even so, I grew more and more edgy during the trip. Michael suggested we turn around and go home, but I wouldn't hear of it. I'm close to Lynette, the sister we were going to visit, and my mother had come down from Pennsylvania to help out in whatever way she could. Knowing this, Michael chose not to argue with me. Being with my family helped to calm my fears and I could enjoy the recital.

That evening, after the recital, we all went to church. As we approached the building, I began to feel a great urgency to get inside as quickly as possible with my baby. Though I could not have said what the threat was, I was certain we were in imminent danger. I didn't try to explain my fears to my husband or family; I simply quickened my steps and began to walk ahead of them. "Let's go, we have to hurry,"

I said. Maybe they thought I was simply concerned about being late. Whatever the reason, they hurried to join me. We entered the church and found a pew in which we could all sit together.

The service began, and I let the music soothe and relax me. I felt safe until the choir finished singing. Then, my fears began to return and I grew increasingly uncomfortable. The church was no longer a sanctuary to me.

At first, I couldn't understand why. Then, I saw it. When the priest prepared for communion, I saw him set up a second altar—one clearly arranged for a human sacrifice. I couldn't believe what I was seeing. I looked around and it was as if no one else even noticed. No one was going to stop this blasphemy. Then, I began to pay attention to the words the priest was saying. I couldn't catch them all, but I heard "devil" and "blood" clearly, and I could follow enough of what he was saying to know he was talking about a blood sacrifice. He was preparing to sacrifice my baby. I watched him pick up the basin designed to catch blood from the sacrifice and move to stand before the evil altar.

I saw that there were two lines of people heading towards the front of the church. On the right, there was a line of happy, smiling people. On the left, was a line of solemn, grim people and they were heading for the sacrificial altar. Ushers directed members of the congregation towards one or the other of the two lines. I knew I couldn't stay where I was. My family was being directed towards the sacrificial altar.

I don't remember exactly how I managed to leave my seat and make it to the safe side of the church, but I did. I found a seat in a pew up front, close to the safe, communion altar. I knew that I had to protect my son and I drew spiritual power from it.

While people were still standing after communion, I lifted my baby above my head, towards heaven, and cried out, "This is the Son of God." An enormous sense of relief and peace swept through me. I had placed my son into a protection the evil force that beset me could not violate.

There was complete silence in the church. No one spoke a word. Then, the service resumed as if nothing had happened. I sat in the pew and held my baby. Slowly, the power that had filled me dissolved and I grew cold. I began to shake.

The service ended normally and people began to leave. A kind, older woman approached me. She took my hand and pressed some money into it. "Take care of yourself, dear," she said. I had no idea why she'd chosen to do such a thing, but her compassion and concern were evident. Alone in the church, I felt safe and did not want to leave.

I began to wonder where Michael and my family were. I would learn later that they were speaking with the police and others outside the church. After a while, Lynette came back inside, looking for me. My mind cleared as soon as I saw her, and I was able to leave the church with her. She took me to her SUV and I began to breastfeed my baby. Her husband, Bruce, was in the driver's seat and had the engine running. I sat there, nursing my son, until the police left.

I think now that the female police officer who responded to the call and consulted with my family must have had at least some understanding of what was happening to me. She did not confront me and did not try to force me to put my baby back into the car seat for the drive home. I clearly needed medical help, but terrifying me and forcibly dragging me to the hospital was not the right approach. I held my son and nursed him during the entire hour-long drive home.

Before I left home that morning, I'd put a roast into the slow cooker. Lynette and my mother encouraged me to eat something and fixed me a plate. I sat down at the kitchen bar and took a bite of the roast. Almost immediately, I was overcome with nausea. I could not swallow and had to run for the bathroom. Leaning over the toilet, I began to vomit. Since I'd eaten nothing for hours, I could not imagine why I was suddenly so ill.

From the bathroom, I could hear Lynette, Bruce, and my mother discussing me. "What is happening to her?" my mother asked. They only knew I had been in the hospital; no one had told them exactly what had happened. They were desperate to figure out what was causing my strange behavior.

"She is not in her right mind." That was Lynette speaking and as soon as I heard it, I knew I could no longer trust her. The evil force was in my head now, telling me to trust no one in my family, especially not my sister. "Do not trust them," it whispered over and over again.

But I desperately needed to talk to someone I could trust—someone who might understand what was happening to me. Suddenly, I thought of my pastor's wife. The thought became a compulsion. I had to see her immediately.

Michael and I attended a non-denominational church that met around the corner from our house. I called the pastor's wife and she agreed to see me right away. Michael drove me the short distance to her house, while my mother, Lynette, and Bruce remained at my house with my sleeping son.

I needed peace, comfort, and most importantly, spiritual protection. I didn't think I was ill; I was sure I was under attack by an evil force. So, I began to feel better as we entered the pastor's beautifully decorated home. But, as we started to talk, it became clear to me that he and his wife thought the problem lay with my family. They encouraged me to get away from them for a while. I felt my muscles go rigid with distrust; they seemed to want me to be alone and vulnerable. I wanted to leave the pastor's house immediately.

I stood up to go and no one objected, but no one arose either. "I have to leave now," I said. My husband got up, a little reluctantly it seemed, but the pastor and his wife began to pray aloud for us. That should have comforted me, but it didn't. Their words seemed hollow and frightened me. I moved to the door and Michael followed. It still seemed to me that he was reluctant to go and I was beginning to distrust him as well.

So I made the decision to take my safety into my own hands. As we approached our Jeep, I walked to the driver's side. "Give me the keys," I said. "I'll drive."

Michael refused. He started to explain, to tell me that I was in no condition to drive, but I refused to listen. I insisted and he refused again. Then, I—a person who had never, ever physically attacked another human being—kicked my husband in his crotch.

It was a horrifying moment. What had I done? Had the evil force won and completely possessed me? Everything seemed to stop around me. I don't remember Michael's reaction or exactly what happened next, only that my pastor, who must have heard the commotion from inside his house, was now standing beside me. He began to pray aloud. It was probably the only thing he could think of to do, but for some reason I found it terrifying. I began to shake all over. My mind was racing with thoughts I couldn't control and I wanted to get away from him, from my husband, from everyone I knew. The whispering in my head had started again. "These people are evil. Do not trust them," the voices said over and over again.

I started pacing back and forth on the sidewalk. I wanted to leave, but since Michael still had the keys I had no transportation. I felt trapped and surrounded by danger. *"In the name of Jesus, I rebuke you."* I repeated this over and over to myself. I wasn't entirely sure who or what I was addressing. My husband? My pastor? Or something much worse and nameless from which there was no earthly defense.

The neighborhood around me was quiet and dark. The streetlights were placed at long intervals and the houses, though brightly lit, were set back from the street. Still, I thought there was a chance someone could hear me. There was a chance I could summon help.

"Help me! Please help me!" I screamed at the top of my lungs, over and over again. I wanted to make as much noise as possible. Even through closed windows and over the blaring of televisions, someone must be able to hear me, I thought. But none of the doors on the street opened. No one came to my aid. The only movement I saw was my husband standing at the pastor's front door. He was talking on the telephone. I continued to scream for help, sure now that time was running out for me.

The police came, and two officers handcuffed me and forced me into the back of their police car. I was 29 years old, married, the mother of a small child, and had never had anything more serious than a parking ticket. Now I was living my own episode of *Cops*. I was terrified. *"In the name of Jesus, I rebuke you. In the name of Jesus I rebuke you."* I whispered it over and over to myself. I badly needed something to hold onto, some power of my own to claim.

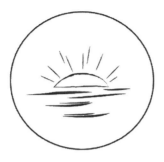

Chapter 3

The Terror Has a Name

I remember almost nothing about my admittance to the hospital. From my perspective, I woke up to find myself a prisoner again. Once again, I was told to take medication—a clear liquid—but given no explanation as to what it was for. This time though, I was carefully observed. The nurses made sure that I swallowed each dose. I suppose I must have told my husband I hadn't taken the medication when I was in the hospital before. He would have explained that to the doctor, of course.

That seemed, at the time, like the ultimate betrayal, but I had no choice. Alone, friendless, and as terrified as an orphan child, I did everything I was asked to do. I wanted the confusion to stop. I wanted the fear to end. I wanted to go home. I wanted to see my child.

Years later, as I write this book, I have access to my medical records from this period. The doctor who had seen me during my first hospitalization had added a note concerning my discharge and subsequent re-admission.

> *This patient apparently was seen and medically cleared by me on her discharge in early February. The patient had no previous psychotic breaks. She had been medically stabilized and discharged. I even had a Rorschach (test) done in the chart to see if she was presenting with symptoms of psychosis. She really reconstituted almost immediately. It is my understanding though now, after the fact, that she was apparently cheeking the medicine. Nevertheless, she reconstituted; she was clearly not psychotic at the time of discharge.*

The doctors told me that I would have to stop breastfeeding my baby. This time the medications were stronger, and it was already clear I would be taking them for a longer period of time. I was devastated. Breastfeeding had been going well for me, and I believe that, if possible, breastfeeding is much better for an infant. And with everything else that had happened, it seemed like the only thing at which I was still succeeding. Now, I felt like a total failure as a mother. Once I stopped breastfeeding, my monthly cycle returned almost immediately and, with the hormonal changes this caused, my emotional state deteriorated further. How on earth had I gotten to this point?

It was now late February 1996, and my precious baby son had been born about a month before Christmas. He came into the world ten days before his scheduled due date and caught us not quite prepared. The first week of his life was a whirlwind.

I was exhausted and sore from the 26-hour delivery and Michael changed more diapers than I did, but already the love I felt for this tiny, newborn human being was like nothing else I'd ever experienced. I love my husband. I love my parents. I love my family and friends; but the immediacy and intensity of this love took me by surprise. No one can adequately explain it or prepare you for what it will be like. The first time that I took my son into my arms, my priorities changed forever. He was completely dependent on me for everything, and I knew I would do anything I had to do to be there for him.

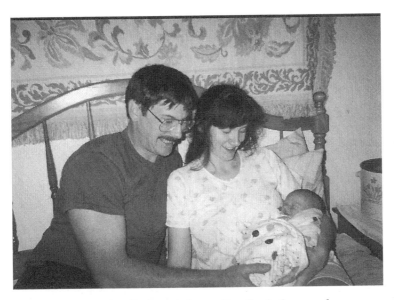

My happy new family just 4 days after the baby was born

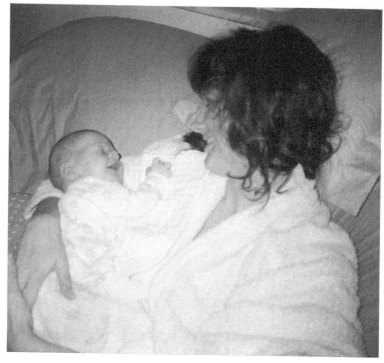

I was tired but at 2 weeks postpartum, I felt bonded with my baby

I did expect the "baby blues," though. My sister, Lynette, who had gone through childbirth twice, had warned me, "Be prepared; you may cry for no reason at all, but it will pass in a few days." Most mothers experience this, and my symptoms were fairly typical—exhaustion, weepiness, and painful breast milk engorgement.

By the end of the second week after delivery, though, these had subsided. The weepiness passed in only a few days; Lynette had been right on the mark. With rest, my exhaustion faded and my body healed quickly from labor, the episiotomy, and the delivery.

My son had taken well to breastfeeding, and was growing and gaining weight rapidly. I remember how complimentary the nurse was at his two-week checkup. "Your son is doing very well," she said. "Most breastfed babies do not usually gain weight quite so fast."

I smiled with quiet pleasure. My son weighed eight pounds, seven and one-half ounces at birth and, already, he'd gained a pound and grown two inches. As a first-time mother, I was delighted and reassured to see that I was providing so well for my child. "I am going to be a wonderful, loving mother," I thought. Christmas, only two weeks away, would be even more joyous that year.

I am the youngest of eight children, now grown and scattered about the country. It's rare that all of us can get together at the same time. But that year was special; it had been several years since a new baby was born into our family. On Michael's side of the family, my son was the first grandchild and first great-grandchild to arrive. We planned to spend the holiday with my sister, Danielle, who lives in a big house on the water. My mother, my two brothers and their wives, four of my sisters and their husbands, and all but one of my nieces and nephews were to be there. Only my sister Patricia, who owns a restaurant and finds it hard to get away, would be unable to join us.

I love Christmas and buying presents for my friends and family is usually one of my favorite parts of the holiday. But my son's pediatrician recommended that I keep him away from public places during his first two months. "You don't want your baby catching the flu or a cold so early in his life," he said. Since it was flu season, I agreed completely as I did most of my shopping by mail order. I had an abundant supply of catalogs, and my love of buying presents had never extended to mall shopping for them anyway. My excitement grew with each brightly wrapped gift that arrived.

That year we passed another milestone: Michael and I brought and decorated our first real Christmas tree, even though we would not be home to see it on Christmas Day. I had promised Michael that we'd have a real tree once we had children. Keeping that promise was a pledge to our family's future.

Christmas celebrates the birth of a child, and that year, it felt to me like the whole family had gathered to celebrate our newborn son. Everyone wanted to hold him, of course, and everyone proclaimed him "precious and beautiful." Naturally, I agreed. The Florida sun was warm and bright that Christmas day, but dim by comparison to the love and warmth that filled Danielle's large and beautiful house. I remember praying that every Christmas would be like this for my son.

Under normal conditions the holidays are often stressful, but Christmas and New Year's passed in a joyous blur for me, and in early January it came time for my routine, six-week check-up. My doctor, who had delivered my son, told me that everything looked good. The episiotomy stitches had dissolved and my vaginal tissue had healed nicely. "You can resume your sex life," she said, and I laughed as she began to sing, "It's going to feel like the first time." She warned me that sexual intercourse would be uncomfortable at first and gave me a sample of vaginal lubricant in case I should need it, but I was not concerned. My son was healthy, happy, and a joy to raise. I was healthy and had been cleared by my doctor to resume normal activity, and I had a loving husband and a healthy marriage. I felt like

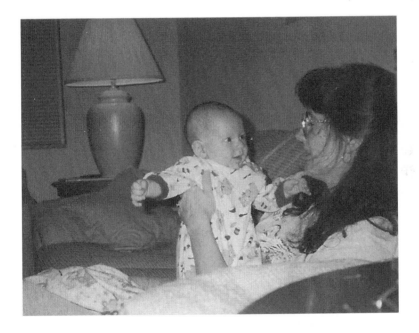

The bond was strong and the love I felt for my baby was immense at 4 weeks postpartum

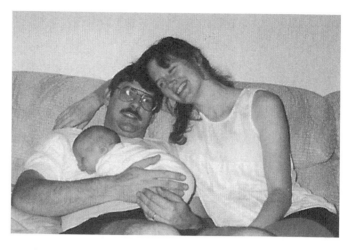

Despite some normal exhaustion, Michael, our son and I were doing fine at 4 weeks postpartum

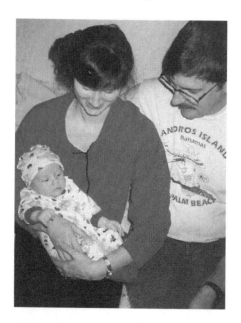

Michael, our son and I in early 1996 after the holidays but before any sign of postpartum psychosis struck

singing myself as I left the doctor's office. I remember thinking, "What more can I possibly ask for?"

When my beautiful, contented baby started sleeping through the night at about the same time, I thought my question had been answered delightfully.

I had planned to return to work twelve weeks after my son was born. I had five weeks of paid maternity leave and planned to take an additional seven weeks of unpaid leave. This is fairly typical for working women in the United States. Most new mothers return to work in six to 12 weeks after giving birth. But I had carried this child for forty weeks. Twelve weeks began to seem like an absurdly short period of time to recover and care for him. Already, he was developing quickly, and I didn't want to miss any of those first, precious milestones.

By the time my son was 6 weeks old, I knew that I would not be able to leave him at a daycare center and return to work. I had been a program director for an occupational health program and enjoyed my professional life. But now I had a new, completely absorbing job and a sweetly demanding boss—my tiny, beloved child. No other job, no career, was ever going to be as important to me as this was.

I was fortunate to have some options not available to many women. I'd planned very carefully for the future and, for several years before I got pregnant, had been able to put most of what I earned into a savings account. This money, I thought, would allow me to take time off from my career to care full-time for my baby. My boss and I had been discussing the possibility that I could work from home for a while, but by now I had decided that this split focus would not work for me. I notified him that I would not be returning to work. A father himself, he understood completely.

The first tiny ripples in my happiness occurred about this time. My son had begun to sleep through the night at 6 weeks, but I could not. The first time he slept all night, I was awakened in the early morning hours by the discomfort in my breasts. Not wanting to wake Michael, I quietly left our bedroom and went into the baby's room, a short distance down the hall. I leaned over the crib to look down at my peacefully sleeping son and gently placed my hand on his belly. "So sweet," I thought, as I felt his breath rise and fall. He was in a deep sleep and didn't stir. I quietly left his room and went into the kitchen, only a few steps down the hall.

My breast pump was on the counter and I took it with me to the kitchen bar. There, with only the stove light glimmering, I placed the breast pump over my left breast and began to squeeze it in and out to extract the milk. It didn't take much, only an ounce or so, to relieve the pain and discomfort, and I moved on to my right breast. Once I'd finished, I discarded the milk. My supply of breast milk had always been more than adequate, and on the occasions we'd tried it, my son would not drink from a bottle. Since I loved breastfeeding him, this hadn't bothered me. The early weeks of his life had persuaded me that I would have no trouble handling the demands of breastfeeding. There seemed no reason to consider other options for feeding him.

I simply modified the nighttime routine I'd established with my son's birth. I'd awaken in discomfort, check on my son, and then go into the kitchen to breast pump. My body seemed to be functioning very well on far less sleep than I'd required before I became a mother.

The seven or eight hours of sleep I used to need to function were becoming a distant memory, and as January progressed, chronic sleep disruption began to take its toll. I noticed it in small ways first. I was edgier and unusually tense. Lack of sleep slowly whittled away my patience, especially with my mother.

Looking back now, I can see that the first major warning sign was a trivial argument with Mom. She and I have always enjoyed an especially close relationship. She was my hero who raised eight children on her own when my father left their 22-year marriage. I loved and respected my mother. I hadn't argued with her or yelled at her since I was a teenager.

On the evening before she was scheduled to return to her home in Pennsylvania, Mom made a comment to me about the checks I was using to pay our bills. Normally, I would simply have laughed or made a comment of my own. That evening, I reacted harshly and started an argument that culminated with me shouting, "Shut the hell up!"

I am normally a kind, loving, patient person. I don't yell at people. The idea that I would shout at my mother, who'd spent weeks as my full-time, live-in helper, astonishes me even now. I was beginning to unravel.

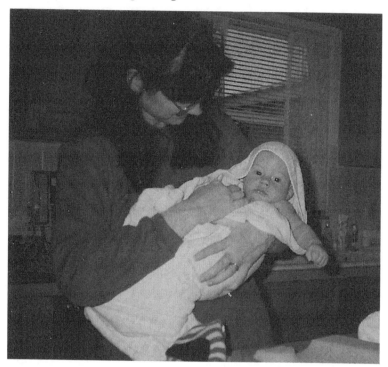

Enjoying bath time at 6 weeks postpartum.

Even then, I recognized that my conflicted feelings about my mom's departure were partially to blame for the argument. Michael had been a wonderful father from the beginning. He loved to cuddle and hold our son, and he was an enormous help when we brought the baby home. But this was a first for him, too. He was still learning "the ropes of fatherhood," and though he helped me to care for our son when he was home, Michael had to return to work as an aviation mechanic after only a few days. Mom had stepped in to help as I healed and grew more comfortable with my new responsibilities as a mother. Once she left, she'd be over eleven-hundred miles away from me. I knew I'd miss her help, her company, and the comfort of experience she brought. Part of me wished she could stay; part of me was ready for her to leave. I knew I was ready to do it on my own.

What I didn't yet see was that it wasn't one quarrel or simply lack of sleep; I was beginning to act in ways far outside my normal character. On weeknights, Michael got home at 11:30 in the evening. He'd worked this shift for many years and I had always been comfortable with it. Once my mother left, though, I became increasingly fearful as night fell and I was alone in the house with my infant son. Suppose someone broke into the house? What if someone tried to kidnap my son? I knew these were wildly exaggerated fears. It didn't matter. My mind created a new list of "what ifs" each night and all the reasoning in the world could not dispel them.

When I decided not to return to work, my happiness had seemed secure. I had never considered the possibility that making a major life decision could affect my emotional state in unexpected ways. With my mother's departure, however, the reality of full-time motherhood had set in. I was now responsible not only for caring for my child, but for doing the laundry, shopping for groceries, planning meals, and everything else involved in running a household. I have a strong organizational background and thought the skills I'd developed in my professional career would transfer well to motherhood. But they didn't seem to do so, and to make matters worse, I quickly realized that most of my friendships and my support network had been rooted in my career life. These were now unavailable. None of my extended family lived close enough to offer practical help and company on a daily basis. The isolation I was beginning to feel intensified my night fears.

I no longer felt safe. Now, when I got up to breast pump, I wasn't simply checking on my son. I had to make sure he was still breathing. No matter what I told myself, the thought that he had died haunted me.

One evening in late January, I sat down at the kitchen bar to write letters. I still owed some thank-you notes from the holidays, and I was looking forward to writing a long letter to a college friend who lives in Greece. I'd always liked keeping in touch with her, and that night it seemed a particularly welcome balm for the isolation I'd been feeling.

I'd just started my letter when I was suddenly overcome by the strong feeling I was about to die. I had no wish to die and no reason to believe my life was in any danger, but I couldn't shake the feeling or control it. Instead, it rooted itself in my mind with the authority of an oracle. I didn't hear a voice or have a vision. I had no idea how my death would come or when it would happen. But I was certain it would come. The premonition was strong and seemed inexorable. I would die and there would be nothing I could do to prevent my death.

I was terrified and overcome with grief. I'd longed for this child and now I would never see him grow up. I'd never get to experience his graduation, or watch him get married, or hold my own first grandchild. And he would never really know me. He would never come to know the person his mother had been. He would never know how much I loved him.

Unless I left something behind to tell him how I felt. "If I am going to die," I thought, "I will leave my son memories of me." Before he was born, I'd bought him a book called *Precious Moments Bible Promises*. Inside are verses from the Bible arranged under headings such as "Promises of Blessings." I opened it and wrote on the front page, *"You should always remember God's promises through it all! Mommy started reading this book to you when you were almost 8 weeks old. I think you understood me even then. I saw it in your eyes."* In his baby book, I wrote, *"Mommy loves you; Daddy loves you; but more than ever, always remember that God loves you! Love Always & Forever, Your Mommy!"*

As I wrote, a feeling of peace came to drive away my fear. "Maybe things will be okay," I thought to myself. I told no one about what had happened, and the next day I kept busy and was able not to focus on the fear. But as soon as night fell and I was alone, it returned in force. The fundamentals of my life were changing quickly in ways I could not have imagined.

By now, I'd added an impressive array of symptoms to my collection: confusion, agitation, false beliefs, paranoia, mood swings, and the inability to sleep. I'd just spent an evening preparing for my own death, and still I hadn't asked for help or even told anyone what was happening to me. I was clinging desperately to "normal."

I remember the evening I spent writing notes to my son in vivid detail, but almost nothing about the night that followed. I know I tried to sleep; I remember lying in bed, waiting for sleep to come. But I was also sure that someone was coming who would harm me and take away my son and that I must not tell anyone what was happening. So, all I could do was lie in bed and wait for the stranger, hoping I would be able to protect my child alone.

He never came and I buzzed through the next day, my third, without any sleep at all. But by evening, I was too terrified to let my husband hold his infant son. Michael was unsure of what to do or how to help me. He decided not to go into work that night and to call Dianne, who was not only my close friend, but had a degree in psychology as well. She had moved back to our town only that week.

I remember sitting in my rocking chair in the living room, protectively holding my son, as we talked. Back and forth I rocked, as if this could save us. But I knew it wouldn't. The danger was all around us and there was nothing I could do. Nothing anyone could do. Dianne sat at my feet and asked gentle questions to help me describe what was happening to me. "How are you?" she asked. "What are you feeling?"

But I had no words to describe the massive fear inside me, even to her. Even to my husband. I was petrified, but all I could do was reminisce with Dianne about our college days and share memories of our friendship. I must have seemed calm on the outside; inside my mind was racing in terror. I couldn't break through the walls of my own facade; I was unable to tell anyone what was happening to me. I had never been so alone.

I don't know how long she and I talked. Perhaps it was an hour, perhaps much longer. I had no real concept of time. I think now that she was patiently trying to help me break through the barriers that isolated me, but at some point during the conversation, I saw Michael leave the living room and go into the garage. He stayed away for perhaps twenty minutes and my distrust of him grew with every passing second. Much later, I would learn that he'd gone to telephone for additional help for me, but what I remember from that night was the growing certainty that I could no longer trust him. He was part of the danger to me and to my son.

Soon after he returned, the phone rang. Michael answered it and passed it to me. It was my doctor, and for a moment I was weak with relief. She would know what was happening to me and what kind of help I needed. "I'm so scared," I whispered, and she immediately offered to come out to the house to see me. I felt like a drowning person offered a life preserver and began to give her directions, only to discover I couldn't. My concentration was now so poor I couldn't put the sentences together. The information was locked up inside me—inside the prison my mind had become.

Michael offered to help, but I wouldn't let him. He, the man I loved and to whom I had been married for the last seven years, was the enemy now. "There is no one I can trust but my doctor," I said to myself. "She is the last chance I have."

Finally, Michael gently took the phone from me. "No, no," I screamed. "You can't talk to her." I was devastated. Now there was no one to trust. I was sure the man I'd loved my entire adult life, the loving father of my precious baby boy, would cut off my last chance for help.

Maybe you've wondered what you would do if everything and everyone you loved were threatened. What would you do if your own life were in danger? I'd thought about things like that, of course; I guess that most people have from time to time. I always imagined, though, that I'd bravely defend myself; that I would be able to fight for those I loved. I had no idea what helpless terror was like. Maybe it's something you can't really understand unless you've been there.

In my extremity, though, I found I did have one thing left, after all—my faith in God. I saw suddenly that I was engaged in a battle against an unseen evil force, a spiritual presence. Only my inner spiritual strength could help me defend my son.

A psychiatrist or a psychologist would call this a false belief or a delusion; to me, the evil force was a very real, very deadly, adversary. If I let go of my son, even for an instant, it would claim him and kill me.

I remember a moment from that terrible night with precise clarity—as though it were a photograph stored in my mind. In it, Michael stands in the kitchen. Dianne is sitting on the couch in the living room. Both are looking at me with concern. I can see it clearly in their faces now, though I couldn't recognize it at the time.

I had been sitting on the sofa as well. Then I rose, holding my son and standing straight and tall, as if preparing for battle. The already brightly lit living room seemed to grow even brighter around me. Our house had an open design, so I could see clearly into the kitchen. I faced Michael, determined to protect our son. I had one weapon. I knew the word of God would help me gain victory over my panic and fear, and most importantly, over the evil force that threatened me. I began to chant, "*I can do all things through Christ who strengthens me.*" I repeated it over and over. "*I can do all things through Christ who strengthens me. I can do all things through Christ who strengthens me.*" The passage seemed to create a shield around us that grew stronger every time I said it. *"I can do all things through Christ who strengthens me. I can do all things through Christ who strengthens me."* I hoped it would be enough to protect my infant son from harm.

Other people began to arrive at our house. They were strangers to me and brought me no comfort. They invaded my home and increased my suspicions. The evil presence that threatened me had flesh and blood allies. I kept chanting. *"I can do all things through Christ who strengthens me. I can do all things through Christ who strengthens me."* I ignored the saliva building in my mouth and began to chant more loudly. *"I can do all things through Christ who strengthens me. I can do all things through Christ who strengthens me."* The strangers did not leave. I had to continue chanting to protect my son.

One of the strangers came up beside me and placed his hand on my son's head. Despite the gentleness of the gesture, I knew it was a deception. He was part of the plan to kill me and take my baby. They all were. Every action gave them away and confirmed my belief that I should trust no one. I had to escape them. I had to escape the gripping fear that consumed me. But how? I saw no way out. All I could do was continue my chant. *"I can do all things through Christ who strengthens me. I can do all things through Christ who strengthens me."*

After three sleepless nights, my senses were as keen as a blind person's. I heard someone say very softly that my doctor had arrived and was outside. The strangers had left the front door to the house open when they arrived, and slowly, slowly I moved towards it as I chanted. I got close enough that I could smell the brisk air. I scanned for people standing outside.

I saw my doctor, walking towards the front door. At least I saw someone who resembled her. All the physical features were right, but every other sense told me this was another deception. "It's not her," I screamed. "You are not my doctor."

I regretted it instantly. The strangers now knew they could not fool me. Several of them grabbed me. I am not quite five feet, eight inches tall and weigh just about one hundred thirty pounds. Four men tried to pry my son from my arms.

The urge of a mother to protect her child is incredibly strong. I felt a surge of power I had never before experienced. I would not give my son up to the enemy. I would protect him. Men grabbed at my shoulders and legs, but I would not release him and I would not go down. I continued my chant, drawing power from the words. "*All things are possible through Christ who strengthens me.*"

It felt like I struggled for hours, but it must have been only a few minutes. At last, I could feel the strength leave my body. I felt my legs weaken. As I began to fall, the strangers attempted to pull my baby away from me. I would not let go. I knew that if they took him from me, I would never see him again. I continued to resist them and continued to chant. *"All things are possible through Christ who strengthens me."*

I failed. I could no longer keep the strangers from pulling me to the ground. As I fell to the damp concrete on my front porch, my doctor caught my son. She had "delivered" him for the second time, I thought. Two men lifted me and carried me down the driveway to a waiting gurney.

My family was, of course, greatly concerned by my condition. The first hospitalization had been bad enough. Now, I was clearly much worse. They had no idea what was causing my bizarre behavior and mental deterioration, but it was clear to them that I was not responding well to the treatment I was receiving. They decided to intervene and arranged for a second opinion. They scheduled an appointment with a doctor who had much more experience and expertise in mental health conditions.

My father, my husband, and two of my sisters accompanied me to see him. I was released from the hospital for the afternoon and assisted, heavily sedated from the medication, into my father's car. All I remember of the journey is a vague sense of relief. At least I was free, if only for a time, from my prison.

My family members were allowed to see the doctor with me, as I was clearly not capable of making decisions for myself. We all filed into his office and sat on chairs before his large, wooden desk.

He began, almost immediately, to ask me questions. I answered as best I could, and gradually, a sense of amazement began to penetrate the mental fog that surrounded me. How did he know exactly what to ask me? He wanted to know if I was confused, fearful, or worried. I confessed, with relief, to all three.

Then he asked me, "Have you been hearing or seeing things?"

"No," I answered quickly. I couldn't bring myself to tell him about the horrible vision I'd had in church. I didn't want my family to hear it.

But he knew. I'm sure he knew that there were things I couldn't say. I could tell by his questions. He asked a few more and then he gave me perhaps the most precious gift I've ever received.

He told me that I had an illness called postpartum psychosis. What was happening to me had a name. It had happened to other women. I hadn't done something wrong and I wasn't possessed. I was ill and I could be treated.

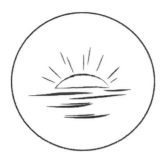

Chapter 4

Treatment Begins

When I was finally released from the hospital, I was prescribed medication that was supposed to take away the fears and bad thoughts I had been experiencing. I took it for the next several months and it did help somewhat, at least initially. Given how horrible I had felt before my admission, almost anything would have helped, I think. But it left me feeling numb and listless. It was as though I was moving through a heavy grey fog and communicating with anyone else, even my husband, was arduous work. I was at ease only with my infant son; we didn't need words to communicate.

The doctor who treated me in the hospital had recommended therapy and referred us to a counselor. Since neither Michael nor I had ever done anything like this, and since we were eager to do everything we could to get our lives back to normal, we simply accepted his recommendation and scheduled the appropriate appointments.

She was a very nice woman, and in another situation I think I might have learned a great deal from her, but the sessions were a mistake. She wanted to focus on our marital relations and had us dredge up past memories and problems in our relationship. I left every session feeling worse than I had when I arrived. Probably the last thing I needed at this point, when I was trying so desperately to understand what had happened to me, was therapy designed to make me question the relationship I considered my rock in a very uncertain world. What I needed, what every woman needs that experiences any mental health challenges associated with pregnancy or childbirth, was counseling from a professional with extensive experience in assisting women with those challenges. I needed to know, to the degree it was medically possible to explain it to me, what had happened to me and what I could expect to happen as I worked to get better. What treatment options were available? How successful had they been in treating other women with conditions similar to mine? What were the risks involved? This was not the time to pursue marital or personal growth, or to solve all of life's problems. I needed practical help to balance my role as a mother with the realities of my medical condition.

And, of course, I needed recognition that it was, in fact, a medical condition. At the time my illness began, our insurance company, like most, separated physical or "medical" illness, from mental illness. Since, by that definition, my problems were not "medical," the company determined that I was entitled only to the very limited coverage its policy provided for mental illness. After that, our quickly dwindling finances were going to greatly dictate how much and what kind of treatment I could obtain.

The only glimmer of hope I saw at this time came from an article my sister Anne and her husband had read in their local paper. It included the story of a woman who went through a serious depression after her child was born, and mentioned an organization called Depression After Delivery, sponsored by an area hospital. Anne contacted the sources listed in the article and was referred to a recently published book called, *This Isn't What I Expected*, by Karen Kleiman. Anne called to tell me about the article, and later she sent me a copy, recommending that I get the book as soon as I could. The conversation and the article itself did help—for two important reasons. First, was the acknowledgement, in black and white on the printed page, that mood disorders after the birth of a child did occur and that there were pro-

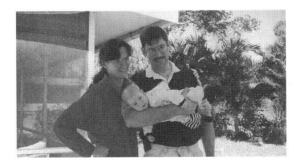

The three of us just one month after the post-partum psychosis diagnosis but before the depression and isolation came upon me.

grams available for treatment. Secondly, of course, this was the story of a woman who had gotten better; it was a ray of light at the end of a long, dark tunnel.

The book itself, though, was less helpful. Part of this stemmed from the fact that reading, during the darkest days of the illness was difficult for me. My concentration had suffered both from the illness and the medications I was taking to treat it. Even more than this, however, was the fact that I could not relate very closely to the woman who had written it. I did not consider myself "depressed," and her experiences were very different from mine. I think the book made only the barest mention of postpartum psychosis. That only added to the sense of isolation I was already experiencing. Slowly, my emotional strength began to slip away again. The medication I was taking was less effective than it had been, and the light at the end of the tunnel seemed even further away.

Then, about a month after I was released from the hospital for the second time, I learned about a support group for women who experienced "baby blues" or depression after the birth of a child. The group met at a hospital near my home, and I was so excited that I registered immediately. More than anything else, I wanted to end the isolation I felt. I wanted to be around people who understood, at least to some degree, what I was going through. Unfortunately, I was going to have to wait several weeks for the next meeting. I needed support now, I thought; I had to hope I could hang on that long. I felt like a desert traveler who had just discovered the next oasis was much further away than it looked.

It was crushing to be so near yet so far from the help I needed, and I almost didn't make it through the wait. About this time, my sleep patterns became disrupted again. By now I was experienced enough with the patterns of my own illness to realize I was on the verge of another major episode. Just as before, my thoughts began to race continually, and my mind was in a state of constant turmoil. I was irritable and plagued by guilt. I didn't simply feel guilty; I was consumed by guilt. I was sure that I was a failure as a mother. It was my fault that our family finances were in jeopardy, and now I couldn't work outside the home to repair them. These accusing thoughts cycled through my mind like a tape on an endless loop. I couldn't shut them off and they added to my intense isolation. I felt trapped in my own house and began to fear that I would have to go back into the hospital.

Then something new happened. Without warning and for no reason I could understand, gloominess overcame me. I wasn't afraid anymore, just so sad I could barely move. No one had prepared me for the possibility that I might move into depression, but even in the state I was in, I noticed that my doctor was not greatly surprised by this turn of events. He prescribed a new kind of medication—he called it an antidepressant—and warned me that it might take a few weeks before it began to help with my sadness. I was becoming an expert at holding on "just a little longer."

I wish someone had told me that women who suffer from postpartum psychosis often experience postpartum depression as well. I wish I had not been left to wander alone in a dark forest full of dangers I couldn't see and I didn't know what to expect. It is important for women to talk to their doctors about what they can expect during the recovery process. They need to ask questions themselves or have a trusted family member ask questions and research their condition on their behalf. The more a woman knows about her illness and the best treatment options available, the better the chance she has to recover completely and more quickly.

But it cannot be left to the patient to begin this dialogue. Neither Michael nor I had any previous experience that would have prepared us to understand what was happening to me. We had no idea what questions to ask, and we relied on our trust that the doctor knew best. There would be a very steep learning curve and many missed opportunities before I knew enough to begin to help myself.

For example, though postpartum psychosis struck when my son was just eight weeks old, he would be five before I learned that there were known risk factors for postpartum mental illness. In my case, these included an earlier miscarriage, a long and difficult delivery, the fact that I grew up without my father, and the stress of being a career woman who always wanted to do her best and please everyone around her.

The biggest risk factor, of course, is a disorder related to a previous pregnancy, though any personal or family history of mental illness increases the risk. I had not had a previous disorder, but the depression I experienced after my miscarriage may have increased my risk. On the other hand, there is no known history of mental illness in my family.

Our knowledge about mental illness related to childbearing is imperfect and still evolving, and there are cases in which a woman with no known risk factors at all becomes ill, but women need access to what is known about illnesses of this kind. Knowledge can ease fear and enable a woman to participate in making informed choices about her own care.

One night, soon after I started the new medication, I was getting ready for bed when I began to have trouble breathing. My heart began to race in my chest and I couldn't sit still. I had never experienced anything like this before and it terrified me. I managed to catch my breath long enough to call my doctor and explain what was happening.

"You are having a panic attack," he said. I had never heard of this before, but it sounded like something that could land me back in the hospital. I could barely breathe and I felt like I might pass out and die at any moment, but the prospect of going back to the hospital seemed worse to me than any of this. My doctor walked me through the attack and taught me a few basic techniques to control my breathing. I was able to make it through the night, and the next day he adjusted my medication once again.

I was—and am—grateful for his calm, reassuring help when I needed it, but now it occurred to me that I was alone in the dark once again. I had no idea that some women with postpartum depression or psychosis experience an anxiety so great that they suffer from chest pains, a racing heartbeat, trouble breathing, or numbness or tingling in their arms and legs. I'd been convinced I was having a heart attack

Surprisingly, despite the medications I was taking, I was still able to drive. I had to force myself to get into the car though; my anxiety made even a trip to the grocery store a major challenge. But getting out of the house, even for short periods, did help ease my sense of isolation, and slowly my sleeping patterns began to improve. With adequate sleep I began to feel better as well, and my medications were decreased. My most troubling symptom at this point became my inability to sit still for any period of time. Later I would learn that this is a side effect of the anti-psychotic medication I was taking.

Finally, the day of the support group meeting arrived. I remember hoping as I drove to the hospital that I would finally meet someone else who had experienced postpartum psychosis. I was desperate to talk to someone who had been through something like what had happened to me; someone who knew what it was really like. I clearly remember the moment when my hopes were dashed. I eagerly pushed open the door to the meeting room only to discover that the room was nearly empty. This was a new group and I was the only mother who had registered to attend the meeting.

The professional counselor who ran the group did have experience with counseling women who experienced depression after childbirth, so I told myself I had made a useful contact. But in the absence of another mother with whom I could share experiences, my excitement had faded and guilt came flooding back. "Maybe I'm the only one," my guilt voice whispered. "Maybe no one else has ever had such a horrible experience after having a baby." I can't remember ever feeling more alone than I did at that moment.

Still, I thought maybe I could see the group leader for individual counseling. She did have more direct experience than anyone else I had met in the area. That, at least, would be something positive. My hope lasted until the next day, when I discovered that since she was not an approved provider, my medical insurance would not cover our sessions. If I wanted the benefit of her experience, I'd have to pay for it myself.

All that came from the experience I'd longed for was that my anxiety deepened. Fearful thoughts began to take over my mind and I began to have trouble speaking. My doctor adjusted my medication several times, trying his best to help, but I was slipping into despair. I could barely remember what it was like to feel well.

My son turned 7 months old in June. He was happy, healthy, and growing fast. I delighted in him, but was troubled by my continuing guilt. I was sure I was a terrible mother and that he deserved so much better. "How sad," I would say to myself, "that his mother is an invalid."

I'd limped through spring barely holding myself together, but now Michael, my family, and I decided that a change of scenery might be good for me. We made plans for me to spend some time in Pennsylvania with my mother and sisters. My son would get to see his grandparents and aunts, and they could provide me with extra support.

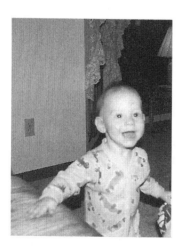

Despite my repeat hospitalizations and the separations, my son was still a happy baby at 8 months old.

We left home in good spirits and the visit began well. Even now, I don't know exactly why things got worse again, but the death of my husband's grandmother seems to have started the downward spiral. I began to lose sleep again and the old, obsessive worry returned that the people I love would die. I could no longer think clearly and began to have trouble remembering when to take my medications. I tried to take care of my infant son and myself, but simple things became harder and harder to do. I lost track of things easily and my inability to cope increased my feelings of guilt. "How could I be such a terrible mother?" I wondered. Sadness overwhelmed me and I was a shadow of the happy, confident woman I used to be.

As my condition deteriorated, Michael's family was preparing for his grandmother's funeral, which only added to my sense of guilt. It was decided, by whom I can no longer recall, that my in-laws should care for my son for a while. They were to pick him up from my sister's house, where we were staying, and the night before their expected arrival, I couldn't sleep. I was tormented by the thought that his grandparents could care for my son better than his mother could, and the conviction that something terrible was wrong with him. Frequent checks did nothing to lessen my anxiety, and I was terrified by the prospect of our separation. What would happen when I was no longer there to protect him? At the same time, I could not sit still and I desperately wanted to get out of the house. I was sure I would feel better if I could just go somewhere else. Where I would go, I had no idea. It didn't matter, just as it didn't matter that it was now the middle of the night. I simply had to leave for reasons I couldn't put into words or even explain to myself. My family tried desperately to calm and comfort me with soothing words and reassuring hugs, but nothing worked for long. Hospitalization was inevitable. I never made it to the funeral.

My husband was due back at work the day after the funeral. Our finances were now too tight to permit unpaid leave, so he was forced to begin the 19-hour drive from Pennsylvania to our house in Florida, without knowing exactly what would happen to me. He was distraught and I was racked by guilt. Without meaning to, I had managed to tear our family apart. Where had I gone wrong? What had I done wrong?

This was my third hospitalization in six months. Though they didn't understand what was happening to me, my family tried desperately to protect me. They wanted to enclose me in safety, but there was none. They tried to encourage me and help me overcome my fears, but I felt like I was drowning in them. It seemed to me that I had failed on every level as a wife and mother, and even a visit from a childhood friend did nothing to lift my spirits. She had given birth to her fourth child about the time my son was born and she seemed to be doing well. I couldn't begrudge her happiness, but it painted a stark contrast to my own misery. I knew she was concerned about me. Everyone was concerned about me. Yet no one seemed to understand what was happening to me. It was as if I'd suddenly started speaking a language that no one around me had ever heard. I could not explain what was happening to me to anyone I loved; the gulf in our experience had grown too vast.

One of the cruelest aspects of an illness like mine is the isolation it creates. Unless they have experienced something similar, no one around you can really comprehend what you are describing—it's all too far outside their experience. I'm told that soldiers returning from combat often feel much the same way when they finally come home.

In an effort to find some explanation for what was happening to me, my family pushed the hospital in Pennsylvania to perform additional medical testing. During my first two hospitalizations, I had nothing more than routine blood work and heart monitoring, but now the doctors decided that I should undergo a CAT scan. They took x-ray pictures of my head. No one told me why the test was ordered or what they were looking for, but of course I cooperated. More than anyone, I wanted to figure out what had happened to me. Any clue they could find might help me get better. But it seemed the results were inconclusive. No further tests were ordered.

My family didn't give up, though. As soon as I was released from the hospital, my sister Anne took me to see a female doctor who specialized in glandular and hormonal disorders. She seemed kind and well informed; she was also the first person to suggest the possibility that my hormones might be out of balance. She ordered new blood tests that yielded some abnormal results. As a result, she recommended hormone treatments and we began immediately.

But by now, I had spent most of the summer in Pennsylvania. I needed to return to my home, and home was twelve-hundred miles away. There was no one in my area to which the doctor could refer me. I felt like I was on a fast moving train that was going nowhere.

71

At home, whatever progress I had made with hormonal therapy melted away, though I still continued to use the cream she prescribed for me. My own doctor did what he could to stabilize me, but his attempts were unsuccessful. By Labor Day, my mental state had slipped out of control again. My confusion had increased markedly and I was convinced that my son was in constant danger. Despite the medications I was taking, the terrifying visions returned. I spent Labor Day weekend confined in the hospital for the fourth time.

With every hospitalization and every separation from my son, my eroded self-confidence slipped further and my guilt increased. I must, I thought, be a terrible mother, a terrible person to deserve this. Thank God my son continued to thrive, but why could I make no real progress? Every time I improved a bit, the downward spiral would begin again and cycle me right back into darkness. In nine months, I had gone from a happy, confident, content new mother to a woman so filled with fear, guilt, and anxiety that I had trouble performing small tasks. Simply taking a shower had become a major effort, and now, for the first time, I had become afraid I would accidently harm my baby or myself. The medications I was prescribed were supposed to help with all of this. Why did they only seem to work for a short while? How did I come to this?

Much later I would learn that the proper balance of medication is critical in the treatment of postpartum psychosis. If the balance is incorrect, many women experience the kind of roller-coaster ride that I did during treatment. This was one more hidden danger in my dark forest.

I was discharged from the hospital after ten days. This time, I had never lost touch with reality, but I left with a deep sadness that I was unable to shake. Once again, my doctor decided to change my medications. By now, he was convinced that there had to be a link between my symptoms and the onset of my monthly cycle. So he discontinued the hormone-related cream the Pennsylvania doctor had prescribed, and he suggested that I add an estrogen hormone patch to my daily routine.

I remember trying to summon up some optimism for the change in regime, but mostly I think I felt a grim determination. This time it had to work. This time I had to really get better. Maybe the doctor actually had found the key to why I could not shake off this illness. Slowly, I managed to recover a little hope, a glimmer of light in my darkness.

Then the letter came. My insurance company notified me that I had now reached my lifetime limit for mental health benefits. Almost immediately, I decided that I would have to go back to work. I couldn't say that I felt substantially better than I had, but even the challenge of balancing work and motherhood was better than the overwhelming burden of guilt and stress I felt over our financial condition. I was unable to find a full-time position, but I did find a fairly good part-time job. For the first time since postpartum psychosis struck, I had regained at least a small measure of control over my situation. That, and the stress relief my additional income provided, helped a bit. I began to feel a little better, a little more like the person I had been.

By the time my son celebrated his first birthday, my condition had improved noticeably. I managed to balance work and motherhood much better than I feared I might. Still, there were signs of trouble to come. My anxieties had diminished somewhat, but they were still present. I worried about my health and the state of our finances. I worried about how my son would fare while I spent my time at work. Worst of all, I was still not sleeping well. I had almost forgotten what pure, natural sleep felt like. The last time I could remember sleeping for seven or eight straight hours was during my pregnancy.

The medications were supposed to help with this, but they never seemed to create the kind of restful sleep I needed. In the morning, when I went to get out of bed, I felt rigid. Some mornings I could barely get out of bed at all. Not so much because I felt tired, though I am certain I actually was sleep-deprived, but because I was filled with anxiety about the coming day. Only my determination to get completely well, to become the woman I had been, propelled me out of bed. Still, I was amazed at what I had actually accomplished and proud of how well I had managed to hold things together.

By the time my son was 16 months old, I was working full-time. My little toddler seemed quite happy in the daycare center at the hospital where I worked, but the struggle for me had become harder and harder. I realize now that the medications I was taking kept me at least marginally functional, but they couldn't do much to alleviate the trauma, guilt, and isolation I felt most of the time. My heart was torn between my desire to be a full-time mother to my son and the necessity imposed by my accumulating medical expenses. That stress increased when the insurance company informed us that they would no longer pay any of my medical expenses. I could see money going out at a much faster rate than I could earn it, even by working full-time. And I was no longer sure that I could continue to do that much longer. I could feel myself slowly losing the battle I'd waged to stay functional and meet the challenges in my life.

What were my options? All I could see is that I had to stay employed to afford any treatment at all. It was my only hope for a full recovery. I could not afford to stay home with my son. If I came to the point that I could no longer work, I would, it seemed, be out of options and out of hope.

All my life I had been a person who knew what she wanted and who tackled life with a smile on her face. Now I seemed pressed by insurmountable difficulties. I had always had a clear, organized mind. I was a planner and I could find my way through challenges that stymied others. Now, I seemed barely able to marshal my own thoughts. I didn't know what to do other than what I was doing. I would do it for as long as I could. I could barely sleep and I no longer knew what it was like to simply relax and laugh.

I no longer recognized the face I saw looking back at me in the mirror.

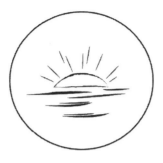

Chapter 5

To Hell and Back

There was nothing unusual in my weekly planner for April 22, 1997. I had entered a number of personal and professional activities throughout April and into May. I marked off a number of holidays and special events, but nothing stands out as I look back through its pages. When I go back and look at my journal for the period, I see that I was actually feeling much better than I had been for some time. So what happened next was completely unexpected.

I remember that my son was ill. He vomited one morning and that is the last memory I have of him for some time. Probably I remember this because his illnesses always troubled me. I always worried they were more than normal childhood ailments.

Perhaps this happened on the morning of April 22nd. If so, he must have recovered quickly because I drove him to his daycare center later on in the morning. I don't remember doing that at all, but I did. I also drove myself back to the house. I don't remember that either.

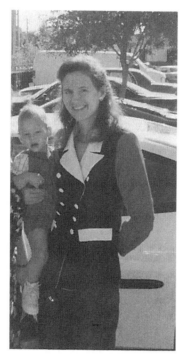

My son and I less than one month before April 1997 when things seemed better and I was back to work.

What I do remember of that day is my growing sense of panic. My mind and heart began to race, and I started to shake with fear. Why, I didn't know. I tried to tell myself there was nothing to fear, but I could not relax physically. I couldn't calm my mind. I could not remember who I had been before this illness took control of my life. All I knew was that I was in terrible danger.

In the midst of all this, I heard a knock on our front door. Rather than answer, I went rigid and silent, barely breathing until the caller had left. Those long moments of waiting escalated my panic to something beyond anything I'd experienced. Now it wasn't just the need-for-safety panic I'd felt when my son was 8-weeks-old. That had been terrible enough; this was a massive, gripping terror that swept away everything in its path. Now I was sure that there was no safety anywhere—

no place to run or hide. It was as though the evil force I thought I'd encountered when I was first ill had returned to invade my home—much stronger, and much more deadly than it had been then. My husband kept a gun in the house and I remember getting it out of its hiding place and finding the ammunition. I tried to load the gun, but panic had claimed me; I couldn't summon enough concentration to control my hands. Now I thank God for that. Disordered as my thoughts were, I was attempting to defend myself; if there was nowhere to run, I would fight instead. Yet, because I was sure I did not face a flesh-and-blood enemy, a gun could provide me no protection. Looking back now, I see how easily terror might have turned a protective weapon into an instrument of escape. Then it was only a puzzle I could not put together. I dropped the useless pieces in despair.

Adrenaline was coursing through my body and every instinct told me to flee, though by now I was sure no escape was possible. Strangely though, I was also overcome with the desire to sleep. I actually remember thinking that if I could just fall asleep, I would be safe. None of this made much sense, even to me, but I was far beyond rational thought and no longer in control of my actions. Despite my confusion, I clearly remember reaching up to the top of the refrigerator to grab one of the bottles of pills I'd been prescribed. Retrieving it, I then opened the door to the refrigerator and looked inside. I found a wine cooler; it must have been there since before my pregnancy. Bizarrely enough at that moment, finding it seemed like a stroke of good fortune. I opened the wine cooler and drank it as I swallowed all of the pills in the bottle.

Then I left the kitchen and went into our master bedroom—the beautiful master bedroom that my husband and I had added onto our house a few years earlier. I knew I had to sleep. I must have changed out of my work clothes because I vaguely remember sitting on the bed in my underwear. More clearly I remember that the phone rang. Slowly, already awkward, I picked up the receiver. I heard my husband's voice. "Is everything okay?" he asked.

Very matter-of-factly I told him what I had just done. This is the last memory I have of the day. Much later, I would learn that Michael had felt a strong urge to call when he had. I believe that was divine intervention. If he hadn't done so, I would not be alive today.

My next memory is very foggy. I lay in what I recognized as a darkened hospital room, and I saw that the person sitting by my bed was a minister from our church. The memory is like a still photograph; there is no sense of time associated with it. Then, or maybe much later—I have nothing to judge this by—I remember seeing red, blood red, in slashes of color. Imagine watching someone slash into a painting with a knife. Now, in your mind's eye, take away the knife, the arm that slashes, and the painting. Only the motion remains and that is as close as I can come to describing what I saw.

I heard terrible screams as well. I looked around trying to see who was screaming, but I saw only the violent red slashes. I felt no pain at all, so I was sure that the screams were not coming from me. I don't know how long this experience actually lasted, but it seemed to go on forever. I remember trying, quite calmly, to figure out who was screaming so horribly.

Next, out of nowhere, I was lying in a hospital bed in a hallway. A woman approached the bed and I remember nothing more for some time. Then, somehow, I was sitting in a chair with a tray of food in front of me. The tray was attached to the chair. I remember trying to get up out of the chair, but I couldn't. I didn't have the strength to lift myself, no matter how hard I tried. And I tried hard; I'm sure of that. Two women came over to settle me back into the chair. I couldn't speak to them; I couldn't tell them that I wanted to get up. I was weak and trapped in the chair, unable to move. I don't remember ever getting out of that chair.

At some point though, I must have done so, because the next thing I remember is being forced into a room without any windows. My captors—and that is what they were to me—gave me a shot and left me lying on a padded floor all alone. I saw the door close behind them and I lay quietly until my breathing returned to normal.

Now, at last, I knew where I was. I was certain I had died and gone to hell. Even if I'd had the strength to stand, there would be no way out of the room in which I was trapped. I would be there forever, I thought, and no one would ever be able to hear my cries for help. It was the only possible explanation for what was happening to me. But what had I done to deserve this?

Then the door slowly began to open. There was no one there; it just seemed to open by itself. And it stayed partially open. I was too terrified to move; too frightened of meeting whatever force had opened that door. Suddenly my prison, awful as it had been only a moment before, seemed like safety.

I don't remember how I came out of the padded room, but I did, of course, and now I began to realize that I was actually in a hospital. That helped calm me; at least my situation, though dire, was comprehensible in human terms. Up to that point, I had seen almost no one and had interacted only, if briefly, with the two women who had settled me back into the chair. I was relieved now to see that there were other people around me.

They appeared to be patients in the hospital as I was. I remember one young woman in particular. She wore glasses and she was crying, saying over and over that she was in pain and suffering. I don't know what she suffered from and no one came to her assistance. There was an air of sad hopelessness that permeated the building and all of its patients.

Not only was it sad, but it was frightening as well. Sometime later, I recall sitting in a room with a group of people. A woman was speaking to the group; she was saying something about emotions, but I cannot recall exactly what it was. Suddenly, I heard a loud commotion and rattling in the hallway outside the door. It frightened me so badly that I could not remain seated. I stood up, ready to flee, when the woman spoke.

"Sit down," she commanded. She was clearly in authority and she spoke harshly. I sat, startled that she'd addressed me in such a tone. After a few minutes, it got quiet outside the door.

These are the only memories I have of the events that occurred after I spoke with my husband on the phone. I don't recall being transported to the hospital, or having my stomach pumped, or having my heart restarted in the emergency room. Each memory of that dreadful place is like a snapshot frozen in time, and hard to relate in sequence to the others. Probably because of the medication I was given, it would be days before I began to understand what had happened to me.

I discovered that I was being kept on the fourth floor, the psych ward, of the hospital where I used to work. One day, as I looked out the window, I recognized an outside area of the building. I had passed it every day for years as I walked down the hallway to my office. Seeing from the inside, where I now was, I was overcome with shame and sorrow. How could it possibly have come to this? I did not know.

One day, as I lay in bed, a man I recognized from work came into my room. He was a primary care doctor, and he told me that he and his partner saw all of the patients on the fourth floor. So now, I would have to see him as a patient. As he turned to leave, he said to me, "I cannot believe you did this to yourself."

The words still pierce my heart and writing them brings back some of the remorse and shame I felt at that moment. I think that only God can know how I felt; it's beyond my power to describe.

Yet even then, sick and confused as I was, I knew there was more to the story. I could not remember much that had happened to me, but I did know, deep in my heart, that what I had done was beyond my ability to control. Even through the remorse and shame, I held onto that. I was ill, not weak, or evil, or culpable. I needed knowledge and treatment, not judgment and contempt. It would take some time to blossom, but something had changed in that moment.

The next thing I remember is sitting in a room with my husband, watching a video on some type of testing. I had grasped this much, but not much more. I couldn't concentrate on what I was seeing and hearing, and was so tired and weak that I lay my head in my husband's lap and let the words from the video simply wash over me. I was unclear what they had to do with me anyway. My ability to speak was still very limited; even if I'd had the strength I could not have asked what we were doing here.

I think it was the next day that I was taken by wheelchair to the basement of the hospital, into an area in which a bed was set up in the middle of what looked like some type of toolbox. The toolbox was large and painted a bright red. I remember being laid flat on the bed and that a doctor I did not recognize came to stand by my head. I heard a buzzing sound and my head began to vibrate. I felt my jaw clench and then there was nothing.

The next thing I remember is being back in my room. The nurse brought a tray of food into me. I was too sick to eat, though, and vomited at the smell of the food.

The routine of being taken downstairs by wheelchair, hearing the buzzing sound, having my head vibrate, and getting sick went on for what seemed like days.

One last memory of my hospital stay involves a hospital worker who came to my room to ask if it would be okay if one of my former co-workers visited me. I had always been a sociable person who loved seeing old friends, but I didn't want anyone I ever knew to see me here. And I certainly didn't want to be seen in the condition that I was in. But my ability to make decisions was so poor that I had to ask the hospital worker for help. He recommended against the visit, so I declined. My brain seemed to ache and I had trouble processing even the smallest thought.

I have no idea how long I remained in the hospital. I settled into a routine of meal times and a few regularly scheduled events—like working on art projects. In truth, I was being treated like a small child rather than a grown woman, and I was beginning to think that this was necessary and appropriate. The hospital environment seemed to encourage such thoughts. I felt I had lost the right to independent action.

When I was ready to leave the hospital, my father asked if I would like to stay with him for a while. He had left my mother when I was a young child, but as I grew up we began to develop a relationship. I agreed to stay with him; at that point I think I would have agreed to whatever anyone proposed. I believed that I could not be left alone to care for myself or my son, so I did not question leaving the hospital with my father. I felt like a walking zombie.

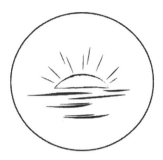

Chapter 6

The Turning Point

My father's house was 50 miles from my home and the hospital from which I just been released. For me, though, the journey was much longer; I was returning to life from a sojourn in hell. As the effects of some of the stronger medications wore off, I began to piece together what had actually happened to me. Much of it I would never remember though and family members had to fill in the gaps for me.

I had spent two weeks in the hospital and during that time I had been given several electroconvulsive therapy (ECT) treatments. These happened in the room with the bright red toolbox, and explained the buzzing sound I remembered and the vibrations in my head.

ECT can be used as treatment in cases of mental illness, particularly severe depression. Essentially, an electrical current is sent through the brain to induce convulsions. To this day, I have no idea how this could possibly help anyone, but it actually can and does help in cases of severe depression or psychosis.

Looking back now, I'm still ambivalent about the ECT treatments I received. They did seem to help, and even my own memories confirm that the hospital made an attempt to ensure that my family and I were able to give informed consent. Clearly, as well, I was in no condition, at least at first, to comprehend exactly what was happening and what the effects would be. I'm actually grateful for this; in the state I was in, the thought of someone shooting an electric current into my brain would certainly have caused me to panic. However, as I began to recover and prepared to leave the hospital, there was no follow-up. It would have been very helpful, and far less frightening, to know that short-term memory loss is a side effect of ECT treatments. I think medical professionals routinely underestimate how important it is for patients to understand what is happening to them.

Initially, my stay with my father went well. One day I was even well enough to go clothes shopping with one of my sisters. Since I had just been in the hospital, I had almost nothing to wear with me, so Marie and I spent several pleasant hours shopping in a local mall. It was the first time in a long time that I'd had that kind of uncomplicated fun.

But being separated from my son and husband was hard—so hard that one night I had a severe panic attack. I wandered around my father's house in the middle of the night, feeling like I would never get better, afraid I would never be able to go home and lead a normal life. After just a few weeks, I found myself back in the hospital.

At first, I was devastated; it felt like just one more heartbreaking ride on the roller coaster to me. But I soon began to notice that things were a little different this time. The doctors I had seen during my previous hospital stays had never seemed to even notice who I was as an individual, and they never seemed to recognize or care that my illness had a specific trajectory. I was a bright, caring, honest woman with no history of mental illness who had suddenly become very ill within weeks of the birth of a child. The doctors and hospital workers seemed to assume that I was a person of diminished capacity, someone who had always been mentally ill or deficient; it always seemed that I had to prove, over and over again, my fundamental competency. More than this, even with all we know about mental health today, it seemed to me that I had to battle against the assumption that not only was I ill, I was ill because I had done something to deserve it, "I can't believe you did this to yourself." Only one doctor had said that out loud; almost all of the doctors I met treated me as though this was a given. There had been days when I just wanted to shout, "I'm not in this hospital because I've been messed up all my life!"

This time I met a doctor who seemed to genuinely care about me as person, and who listened to what I had to say. She was a woman and a mother, so I am sure that this helped us relate to one another. More than this, however, she took what I said into consideration and used it to help design and adjust my treatment. After all, who would know better than I did what was going on within me?

She was not an expert in mental illness related to child-bearing, and she did not have all the answers. What she did have was a keen, professional curiosity, and the kind of genuine concern and kindness that I had not encountered at any other hospital. It had been 16 months since my illness began. Why did it take so long to find this type of care? Well, you could say, "better late than never," I suppose, and I do thank God that I survived long enough to obtain better treatment. The problem is that all too many women don't.

After 20 days of changes to medicine and talking with counselors, I was discharged from the hospital and went to stay with my sister, Marie. While I was in the hospital, she had located an outpatient mental health program near her house that she thought might be helpful to me. Two weeks after leaving the hospital I began to attend the program's classes daily.

A doctor taught the classes in a professional, busi-ness-like manner that I, a business major in college, could relate to easily. Though they did not specifically address issues related to childbearing or motherhood, the classes did provide useful information and strategies to help me deal with the emotional trauma of my illness. This is an ap-proach I had not encountered in any of my hospital stays, and I appreciated being treated like an intelligent, competent person who could understand and even assist in her own recovery. I began to feel a bit more optimistic about my prospects, and worked hard to master skills I needed to cope with my anxiety. I was learning that recovery doesn't happen overnight; it takes time and you have to master each step along the way. But I was no longer simply the passive recipient of a doctor's treatments; I was learning how to heal myself. The light at the end of the tunnel seemed to grow a little brighter.

At the end of July, three months after my life was spared, I "graduated" from the program. I had made a great deal of progress, but there were still struggles. I had started working part-time while I was in the program, but I was still living apart from my husband and son. Since the program was an hour's drive from my home, I continued to stay with my sister, and saw my husband and son only on the weekends.

Now that I had "graduated" from the program, I had a decision to make. I desperately wanted to go home to my own family, but there were important advantages to staying that I had to take into account. I had finally found a doctor who was really helping me; I wanted to keep seeing her. Also, I was working and we really needed the money to assist with the expenses I had incurred. Finally, I was surrounded by family members who could provide additional support when I needed it; if I went home, my husband would have to manage that support on his own. I struggled with the decision, but finally decided that I needed to stay where I was for the present.

I managed on my own for several more weeks before I had to take myself back to the hospital. This time it was a decision that my doctor and I made together. Nothing major had occurred, but I was suffering from confusion and having difficulty recalling things. I now believe that at least some of this resulted from the ECT treatments I had received—a predictable side effect I was still unaware of at this point.

Another struggle for me was that my family and my husband had begun to turn against each other, casting blame at one another. This is not uncommon. Most women who experience any mental health challenges related to childbearing carry a burden of guilt and blame. It doesn't matter that the woman has done nothing to cause the illness; she still wrestles with guilt and blames herself for the disruption her illness causes. Often, the guilt and blame spread outward to other members of the family. They may blame themselves or each other for what has happened. Much of this can be alleviated if the woman and her family have access to the best current information about her illness, and if they receive support from individuals who have been trained to support patients and families.

Unfortunately, none of these resources were available to me or to my family. We had to learn, by trial and error, how to support ourselves and each other through the storm of postpartum psychosis. That took time and experience, and we went through a good deal of heartbreak before we got it right. Among the consequences of this learning curve was that I spent my 31st birthday confined to the hospital for the seventh time since the onset of postpartum psychosis.

After my release, I went back to the day program and began classes once again. I re-visited some of the skills I had previously learned and learned some new ones. My husband and I also began going to counseling again. This time, counseling was appropriate for us. It was specifically targeted to address the problems we were currently facing and some of the sessions included other family members as well. By the time I "graduated" once again, two months later, I was doing well and decided it was time to go back home to my husband and son.

Thank God that most of the income I had earned during the years prior to my son's birth had gone into our savings account. Of course, we hadn't put it into the bank because we thought it might be needed for future medical expenses. After all, we had medical insurance; we thought we were safe from that worry. We had planned to save it for our family's future.

Now it seems like a miracle that the money was there when we needed it the most. I don't know what we would have done if it hadn't been there, and if we hadn't received so much support and help from our family and friends.

Even with all of this though, I still needed to work. I kept the part-time job I had and made the hour-long drive every working day. I also continued to see the doctor I had found. The progress I was making in my recovery easily justified the travel time. Now, for the first time since my illness began, I began to think I would be completely well one day soon.

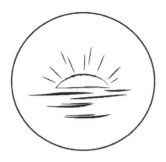

Chapter 7

Process of Recovery

Recovery does not happen because you swallow enough pills—even if they are the right kind of pills. It is a long-term process, with a series of ups and downs, and some very unexpected twists. It requires you to learn, all over again, how to care for your mind, body, and spirit. A major illness changes you; you are not the same person you were before your illness and your needs will be different than they once were; but then, so will your strengths. Usually, the process of recovery uncovers a kind of courage you never knew you had. Discovering that is one of the gifts of recovery, but it often comes at a very high price.

And as hard as the process is for anyone who suffers a major illness, recovery becomes even more difficult for a woman struggling with an illness like postpartum psychosis. Illnesses like this are unusual and most people misunderstand them. Consequently, there is a stigma surrounding illness related to childbearing that adds substantially to the burden of guilt and shame the woman is already carrying.

Every working mother has experienced the pressure of balancing her family and work life, but my illness and our circumstances had intensified these pressures. Like most women who suffer from illnesses related to childbearing, I blamed myself for all of the problems our family faced. It was my fault that there were stresses in my marriage. It was my fault that our financial situation was more precarious than it should have been. Every time my son came down with even the most routine childhood ailment, well that was my fault too. Had I been home with him, it wouldn't have happened. My numerous hospital stays and the time I'd had to spend away from my son meant I had missed a significant portion of his early life, and now I was working full-time again. More blame. Intellectually, of course, I knew this was an overreaction, but that didn't seem to help much. I was still struggling to learn the tools that could help me cope with thoughts like this.

In addition to working, I was still in counseling with my husband, and I was separately seeing a counselor on my own. The sessions were helpful, but they added to an already full schedule. I was having much more trouble coping physically than I would have before my illness, and the pace was slowly depleting my energy and drive.

Things came to a head when my son came down with a stomach virus. It wasn't serious or dangerous, but it started me on the roller coaster once again. Within two weeks, I was forced to check myself back into the hospital once again.

After about four days of treatment, I was able to focus and think more clearly. Reluctantly, I had to admit that I was not going to be able to continue working full-time. The truth was harsh, but it was one that I was going to have to accept. My body would no longer accept the punishing schedule I'd been keeping.

After my hospitalization, I decided that I would look for a part-time job in banking. I had worked at a bank during college and enjoyed it, so this seemed like a promising strategy for me to pursue. Good part-time jobs are not easy to find, and I was overjoyed when I landed a position at a local bank. What I had not counted on, though, was the difficulty I had mastering the new skills I needed for the job. Learning new things had normally come easily to me before my illness; the chance to learn something new and grow had been one of the things that motivated me to advance in my career. It's true that I was sometimes made a little uncomfortable by change—I have a natural preference for order and continuity—but this was easily manageable and probably not much different than the kind of anxiety most people experience. Now, however, change and the necessity of learning new things were deeply distressing. I simply did not have the memory or concentration I once had, and I struggled against my new limitations. I had worked so hard to recover, and now it seemed to me that all the improvement I thought I had made was an illusion. I continued to struggle until it became obvious, even to me, that I would have to go back to the hospital for a few days. At this point, my doctor advised me that I would have to stop working all together.

At the time, that seemed like a devastating defeat. Now, I recognize that it was probably the best thing that could have happened to me. It was time for me to stop pretending that I could go back to the life I had enjoyed before my illness and start designing the kind of life that would help me recover and flourish as the person I now was. I had some serious soul searching to do.

The immediate impact was obviously going to be that our family would have less money without me working. This was the hardest thing for me to accept; I had been determined to work so that we could pay the medical bills I had accumulated. I needed, I thought, to share the burden they imposed on us. It was my husband who helped me change my perspective. "Don't worry about the money," he would say. "God will provide and I'll work more. Everything will be okay." His attitude was, "whatever it takes." It took me some time to believe his words were more than simple reassurance, but his conviction that my health was important helped me reorder my own priorities. I began to let go of the expectations that I now knew to be unrealistic and look for things I could do.

First and foremost, I would be a full-time mother to our son. He was growing up so fast and I had missed so much of his babyhood due to my illness. There was damage to heal;

beginning with the bond between us that had been forcibly broken when he was only 8 weeks old. Even if my energy was not what it had been, I was now much healthier than I had been for most of his short life.

This was the right decision for us. With more of my attention, my son thrived and I found that the pace of my recovery was steadier. I began to feel a sense of joy return to my life. As we moved into 1998, I noticed something else; for the first time in more than two years, I was able to genuinely laugh again.

There were still some rough spots though. Even if I couldn't work, I wanted to make some sort of contribution to the world, and I thought volunteer work might allow me to do that. I could, I thought, make a difference in someone else's life and assist in my own recovery. I decided to attend a training program to become a volunteer at a crisis pregnancy center, but with that decision all the old fears and anxieties came flooding back. It took a great deal of support and encouragement from my husband, but I made it through the program and began to volunteer for the center. In fact, I did well as a volunteer and enjoyed the administrative work I did. For the first time since my illness, I felt appreciated for my contribution and this gave me the sense of accomplishment and confidence I so badly needed. I limited my hours carefully and suffered no ill effects from this addition to my schedule. Other than the decision to stay home with my son, this small step was the first unqualified success I'd had in designing a new life for myself.

Not too much later, I learned that a local, well-known store was hiring. This was a store I loved so much that the prospect of working there was enough to make me revisit my decision not to work at all. Maybe I could get a schedule limited enough to allow me to work there without ill effect. My confidence faltered when I found out that I would have to participate in a group interview to be considered, but once in the group setting something like my old ease and confidence returned. And it paid off; I was offered a position as a "cast member" by the store. I had never had a job that was this much fun.

In the summer of 1998, two and a half years after the onset of postpartum psychosis, my doctor finally took me off the medications I had been taking. I was delighted! I was volunteering one day a week at the crisis pregnancy center and working part-time at a job I loved. It didn't even matter that I wasn't making enough to cover my son's child-care expenses. For the first time since my illness began, I felt like my old self. My mind and body were healthy, and I was happy. That happiness had rubbed off on my husband and son; there's truth in the saying, "If mom isn't happy, nobody is happy." The people who loved me rejoiced to see that I was finally a happy mom.

I was even well enough to resume my exercise program. I had exercised regularly before and during my pregnancy, but not since my illness began. Though I was aware of the benefits of exercise in general, I had never had the energy or motivation to undertake it during the worst of my ill-

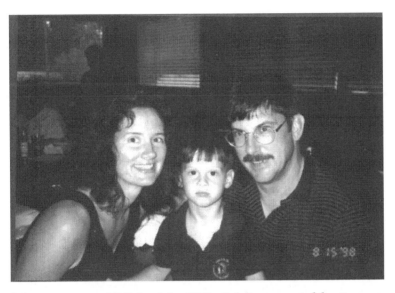

Me, my son and Michael in 1998...I felt recovered by 2 years postpartum when my sense of humor was back by our 10th wedding anniversary.

ness. Nor had any of my doctors encouraged me to exercise regularly. Now, as I felt better, I began taking walks with a friend whenever I could and working out with exercise videos. I learned that not only does exercise keep your body and heart healthy, it increases the "feel good" chemicals in your brain and can help significantly with depression.

Later on in the year, quite unexpectedly, I got a phone call from a manager at the hospital at which I used to work, "We are having a hard time finding reliable help," she said. "Can you do some office work for us?" The job they offered me was part-time, very flexible, and came at the perfect time for us financially. It would help us cover the cost of my son's preschool.

I believe that prayers are answered when the time is right. We don't always see that because we want answers right away. It's when we learn to take steps in faith to meet the challenges of our lives that we are rewarded. I gave up working full-time in order to do what I needed to do to recover. With my husband's help, I was able to put aside my fears about what this would do to our family's finances and trust we could make this work. By doing so, I was able to re-connect with my son to heal the bonds that had been damaged during my illness. I had been so afraid it was too late to fully do that, and I had to fight against the fears and anxieties that arose every time we went through a rough patch. There were times, for example, that my son would not let me dress him. He would kick and cry, and act as though he hated me. Now that I had all the time I needed to spend with him, I could let go of my fear that I was failing as a mother and trust the parenting skills and experience I had gained. All toddlers throw tantrums; they adopt unreasonable behavior and push against boundaries. They learn that those boundaries hold fast and that they are loved anyway. It's all part of growing up for them and parents learn to manage on the job. It amazes me that parents typically begin the most important job they will ever have with so little training.

This joy was not the only reward I received. By the end of the year, I was working two part-time jobs. Both were flexible enough to allow me to work no more than 25 hours a week, and each gave me something I needed. Working in the store increased my self-confidence and helped me redis-

cover fun; working at the hospital made a much-appreciat-
ed contribution to our finances. In a way that I would not
have been able to imagine, what I gave up returned to me,
and in a way that would support rather than harm me.

About this time, I received one other gift. For the first
time, I met another mother who had experienced postpartum psychosis. She came into the store where I worked. She
had brought her baby with her, and that led naturally to
conversation. I asked her the kind of questions one always
asks new mothers, but then I followed up with, "And how
is mom?"

That is a question people often forget to ask. It's natural to get caught up in the wonder and excitement of a
new baby, but mothers need attention they often don't get. I
think the woman needed someone to talk to about her experiences; she began to share her struggles with me. In return,
I shared some of mine and she told me how much it meant
to her to be able to talk to someone who understood. I remembered how much I longed, in my darkest days, to meet
just one person who had been where I was. I didn't know it
yet, but this exchange was the seed of another reward.

We celebrated Christmas with a deep sense of gratitude
that year. In the coming year, my husband and I would
celebrate our eleventh wedding anniversary. We had been
through hell together, but our marriage had survived. We
were still in counseling, but recently we had been referred
to a marriage and family counselor who shared our spiri-

tual beliefs. That turned out to be an important blessing for us. We shared a deep faith in God and were able to fully bring this into our sessions with him. That happy Christmas, as we counted our blessings, we considered that to be an important one. In the coming year it would turn out to be crucial.

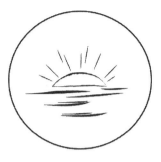

Chapter 8

Trip to the Bizarre

In the spring of 1999, my life seemed to be going very well. I was healthier than I had been since my illness began, and I had every reason to think I'd gotten off the roller coaster permanently. Of course some days were better than others, but I was no longer tormented by the periods of extreme anxiety that had virtually incapacitated me. Michael and I had worked through the stresses my illness had caused in our relationship, and our marriage was strong. We were beginning to plan a family camping trip in Asheville, North Carolina to celebrate our eleventh wedding anniversary.

I was growing in other ways as well. It had become important to me to understand what exactly had happened to me in April of 1997. For a long time after the event, I had been too emotionally fragile and too afraid of being drawn back into the fear to do this. Now I was stronger and I wanted to fill in the memory gaps I still had. I wanted to know what my family had gone through that day. I began to ask questions and my husband and family began to fill in the missing pieces for me. At first they were reluctant—I think they were afraid of causing me new pain—but that changed as they began to understand how important this was to me. I needed to know what had happened, and they took me through that day as it unfolded for them.

For my husband it began when, acting on the instinct that something was wrong, he called me at home. He still clearly remembers the terrible moment when I told him, quite calmly, almost as if I was telling him that I had gone to the grocery story, that I had just taken an entire bottle of pills. He hung up the phone and rushed home from work. On the way, he had the presence of mind to flag down a police cruiser. The officer called an ambulance.

When he got to the house, Michael immediately went to the front door, which was locked. When he tried to unlock the door, the lock broke apart. To this day, we don't know why. Was it simply that there was a stress point in the metal and this might have happened at any moment, or was Michael so full of adrenaline that he applied much more force to the lock than he realized? Whatever the reason, this left only one possible way into the house. There was an outside door that led directly into the new master bedroom. He had to break the storm door handle to get in, but he managed that.

I was lying on the bed. I was still conscious and appeared to be fine. In fact, when the ambulance arrived I was able to talk to the paramedics. This was all reassuring in the moment, but as it quickly became clear that I really had ingested the medication I said I had, the paramedics decided to transport me to the emergency room. Michael stayed behind long enough to telephone my doctor.

Fortunately, the hospital was only a few minutes from our house, because by the time Michael was able to get there, about an hour later, I had already "coded." The doctors told him that they had been able to restart my heart, but I was in critical condition and he wouldn't be able to see me for a while. They assured him that I "should be okay," but all he would be able to do was wait and see.

It was touch and go for me for about three days. I have no memory of any of this except for waking to find a minister from my church sitting by my bed. It's only a brief flash of memory, quickly swallowed up again by the oblivion in which I spent these days.

After I was stable, the hospital arranged my transfer to another hospital with a psychiatric ward. At the time, the decision infuriated my husband and family. They wanted the crisis doctor in charge of my care to transfer me to a different hospital. Their choice was not only located midway between our house and the town in which most of my family lived, it was not a hospital at which I had been employed. They very much wanted to spare me the humiliation of being confined to the psychiatric ward of a hospital in which I was so well known. The doctor insisted, however, and the hospital administrators followed his recommendation. I was admitted to the hospital where I had worked, and placed under the care of a doctor I had worked with professionally.

My husband angrily confronted the doctor about the decision. "I just could not send her to that facility," was all he would say at the time, and that did little to reconcile Michael to his actions. Later, though, we learned there were some things he couldn't say or didn't feel comfortable telling my family. The hospital they had selected had some serious patient care problems. In fact, it had a reputation—at least among health care professionals—for badly mistreating patients confined there. Though his reluctance to explain his reasons is part of a larger problem, the doctor's actions may well have saved my life. For the second time, something unexpected had intervened to change the course of my destiny. I was paying more attention to things like this; fortunate coincidences were beginning to seem far less coincidental.

I was hungry to find a deeper meaning in all that I had been through. Other than the marriage counselor my husband and I were seeing, none of the health care providers I had seen over the last three years had ever suggested that there could be a spiritual aspect to my illness, or that some of the healing I needed might be spiritual in nature. I think that, if asked, most of them, maybe even all of them, would have replied that spiritual considerations lay outside their field. They might well have considered it unprofessional to discuss spiritual matters with their patients; that would not be an uncommon position for physicians to take. I understand the reasons for their reluctance, but I was coming to the conclusion that treating just the physical manifestations of my illness was always going to be incomplete. I needed a more spiritual focus, but was unsure where to start.

My mother helped me take some of my first steps on this path. She and I always had a close relationship; she was my best friend and the person I could talk to about anything. With her I never felt I had to hold back details or thoughts that might upset, frighten, or even scandalize another person. She would simply listen to what I had to say, and she gave me a safe space to begin to talk about my near-death experiences. She could also fill in some of the pieces I was missing, and help me makes sense of the memories I did have.

She told me that various members of my family had been with me in the hospital during the three days I was in critical condition. That was no surprise, of course, but she told me that while my sister, Lynette, was in the room, I regained consciousness long enough to tell her that "I saw Hell and it is a terrible place." I don't remember that Lynette was there, and I don't remember talking to her, but I do remember my fragmented visions of a terrible place.

At about the same time, a neighbor told me something very bizarre about the people who had lived in our house before we bought it. I knew he was a widower, but not much more about him. I remember guessing that he might be selling the house because of the memories it held. I just had no idea how dark those memories were. It turns out that the couple fought continually, and the wife had slipped into drug and alcohol addiction. Finally she took her own life. I hurt for her, but I was also very glad she did not die in our house. Still, it seemed like one more piece of the crazy puzzle my life had become. Could all the anguish they went through have left echoes in the house and could they have affected me? I didn't know then, and I still don't, but I now believe that questions like these are important. How interconnected are we on a spiritual level? Do our souls touch one another across time and space?

All of this was on my mind as I planned for our North Carolina camping trip. Physically I was in the best health I had been since my illness began; if asked, I think I would have said that I was fully recovered—even if not exactly to the person I used to be. I had noticed a few small things over the last year, but they were minor enough that I wrote them off as the normal sort of health variations that trouble people. In the summer of 1998, for example, my period stopped entirely for several months. My doctor never determined the exact cause, and by the end of the year it had returned to normal. Then, in the spring of 1999, I developed a strange looking rash on my ankle. It was not painful and it didn't actually bother me, but I did see my doctor since it persisted. She gave me a cream to apply until it went away, but she wasn't particularly concerned about it. Apparently, it's not uncommon for a rash to appear without explanation, run its course, and then fade away. Now I wonder if I should have paid more attention to it. Was it somehow related to symptoms that followed? I don't think I will ever know the answer to that.

The only real concern I had during this period of time was that I noticed in June that my sleep patterns had begun to deteriorate. I was working at two part-time jobs I enjoyed, and I loved the volunteer work I was doing at the crisis pregnancy center. Best of all, my family life was as happy as it had been before my illness. I had what most would consider a non-taxing schedule in a relatively stress-free environment. But I had learned through bitter experience that sleep disruption was a symptom to which I needed to pay immediate attention. Serious trauma of the kind surrounding postpartum psychosis changes people permanently. I was always going to be especially sensitive to the loss of sleep.

So to be safe, I contacted my doctor immediately. She prescribed me sleeping pills to help re-establish my sleep patterns. Unfortunately, though, I experienced something known as the paradox effect. Instead of helping me sleep, as they were meant to do, the pills actually made the problem worse. To counter this, my doctor wrote me a prescription for a different medication. It was newer, more effective, and known to have fewer side effects. Unsurprisingly, our insurance did not cover it. To this day, I don't know why exactly; their coverage denial seemed like just one more mystifying turn in the medical maze I'd walked since my illness began. But there was no real choice. Sleeplessness is, and was, a dangerous symptom for me. Despite the financial hit, and it was considerable, we paid the full cost of the medication. I was relieved to discover that it worked well and quickly restored my sleep patterns.

A week before we were to leave on our camping trip, I was sleeping well and the doctor and I agreed that medication was no longer necessary. I still had the rash on my ankle, so she gave me a different cream. She had no reservations about my trip and I was looking forward to it. Given what we had been through over the past three years, Michael and I thought this anniversary deserved special celebration.

Our drive to North Carolina is a memory I treasure. We were all elated—glad to be free of our normal routines for a little while and excited by the prospects before us. We were happy just being together and the miles seemed to slip past us. Normally car trips like this are long and exhausting; this one seemed to fly by. It wasn't until we reached the campground in Asheville that things began to change for me. It was slight at first, but slowly I became hyper aware of every detail of the environment around me. I sensed that history here had been tragic and that it had left its imprint on the land, the water, and the people who lived in the area. The river that flowed through the campground seemed charged with memory, and the land seemed ancient and sad. I remembered the story of the woman who had lived in our house. It seemed to me that my near-death experience had left me with a spiritual awareness of discordant energies that I never used to have.

Still, I initially brushed off this awareness; it was not intense enough yet to trouble me and I wanted to have a happy, carefree vacation. I certainly didn't want to open the door to anything like the terrifying visions and sensations I'd experienced during my illness. I wasn't sure where spiritual awareness stopped and psychosis began, and I certainly wasn't ready to find out. As the day progressed though, the awareness had intensified considerably. Now what I sensed wasn't simply sad, or even tragic; it was actively evil. By the time night fell, I felt as if a dark, malignant fog were slowly enveloping us.

That night was bizarre. Despite the evil I sensed all around us, I don't remember feeling any fear. In fact, I remember encouraging my husband to get me pregnant again. Why it was so important right then, I don't know; perhaps it was a life-affirming instinct in the face of danger. My hyper awareness made sleep impossible, but since I had been taken off sleep medication, all I had with me was a natural sleep-aid a friend had given me. It was ineffective and I lay awake in our camper as my husband and son drifted off into sleep.

Alone in the dark, my awareness grew even sharper. Memories of past events played like movies in my mind, and I viewed them with a discernment I'd never previously possessed. The scenes seemed entirely intimate and personal, yet I was as detached from them as if they had all happened to someone else. I saw each event in an entirely new light that seemed profoundly right to me. I let the movies run in my mind until I was distracted by noises outside the camper. Up until then the night had been very quiet; quiet in the way city dwellers never experience until they spend some time in the country. Now, though it was quite late, I began to hear a flurry of activity that seemed localized right outside. Who were these people whose mumbling voices I could hear? Carefully, so as not to disturb my husband, I got up to peer out the camper window. I could see no one; there were no lights and no darker shadows moved through the night. I got back in bed and lay quietly, trying to calm my breathing. Maybe if I was quiet enough they would simply go away. For a moment I thought it had worked. Then I felt the camper move. Something or someone picked it up as if it were a child's toy and began to carry it towards the water. Now I was paralyzed by fear; I could neither move nor speak. I couldn't warn Michael. I couldn't do anything to save us.

As quickly as it had begun the motion ceased. The sounds died away in the night. Slowly my terror began to recede and I began to breathe more normally. While my husband and son slept undisturbed, I lay in darkness and prayed for dawn to come.

The next morning I tried to put the night behind me. In daylight, what I had experienced seemed bizarre and impossible. I couldn't talk to Michael about what had happened; I was sure he'd think I'd been imagining things and he would worry. I still hoped to salvage the trip and give him the anniversary he so richly deserved, and the clarity I'd experienced during the night was gone. Now I was simply determined not to slip back into the nightmare my illness had been. I still had much to learn about the balance between psychosis and spirituality.

All I could do was take one day at a time and I tried to start the day as normally as possible. However, as morning progressed, the night fear came seeping back. Our campsite was near the water's edge and my son was riding his tricycle around the camper. I watched for a while, becoming more and more frightened that he would fall into the water. I tried to coax him to stop riding his bike and do something else, but he was enjoying himself and was determined to continue. Finally, I put my hand on the handle bar and my son let out a yell. He bit me with all the strength in his three-year-old body, every inch the enraged toddler.

Michael, hearing him yell, came running from another part of the campsite to see what had happened. Our eyes met for one long, terrible moment. I'm pretty sure he was afraid I'd done something to cause our son to bite me. The moment passed as he realized he'd walked into the aftermath of a pint-size bid for autonomy, and he began to understand my fear. He tried to reassure me, saying, "It's okay; he's not near enough to the water to fall in." His calm reassurances helped dispel my fear, and we spent the rest of the day relaxing at the campsite.

As the day shaded into twilight, my son and I were reading books together in the camper. A typical toddler, his outrage had subsided as quickly as a summer shower, and we'd spent most of the afternoon playing together. Now, as the sky darkened, my creative 3-year-old came up with a new game for us; he wanted to "search for planets." We shut the curtains that closed off his bed from the main space of the camper, creating a dark, tent-like space. The ceiling became our night sky; a flashlight beam directed into the night became the light from a distant star. We looked for new worlds in this tiny universe and, of course, we found them. I was caught up in the game of pretends and forgot my fears for a while.

After playtime came bedtime. My son wanted me to sleep on his side of the camper, so I curled up beside him and hoped that sleep would come. After missing one night of sleep, I hoped my body would be so tired that it would simply override my active mind. No such luck. As I lay beside my son, the movies in my head started again. This time, though, the scenes I saw had nothing to do with my life. I saw a fire and someone being sexually abused, but it wasn't clear who all this was happening to. Was it my husband? Maybe it was the person who had owned the camper before we bought it. Or perhaps I was seeing images from the campsite's troubled history. Perhaps these were some of the memories that had imprinted themselves into the land and water.

By the time morning came I was convinced I knew what was happening. I was being shown these scenes for a reason; I was meant to help someone overcome something terrible. I could turn someone's darkness into something good. I didn't know how to start or who I was meant to help, but I was sure of my mission. But I couldn't talk to Michael about any of this. I couldn't put it into words I thought he'd understand, and I knew he was already concerned about me. I don't think he expected something major to happen, but he could see I was having problems. Much as I had tried, I hadn't been able to hide this; I couldn't quite act normally enough to reassure him. I realized just how concerned he was when he started packing up the camper. We had planned to stay a week and now, after only three days, he was ready to pack up and leave. When I tried to get him to talk about what he was feeling, my strong, steady husband, my rock through all the storms we had weathered together, finally broke down. "I can't go through this again," he cried.

It broke my heart. He'd shouldered so much of the burden and I wanted more than anything else to give him the respite he needed and deserved. I reassured him that I was fine—and oddly enough despite my night terrors and my sleeplessness, I really was happy where we were—and convinced him to stay. I thought it would be okay. I thought I could keep it together. I didn't realize that things were already spinning out of my control.

Having convinced Michael to stay, I then suggested he take us all to the old airport museum. That was the kind of thing you were supposed to do on vacation, and I wanted ours to get back on track. I thought my son would enjoy seeing the planes and equipment. Michael was reluctant, but he let me talk him into going; he wanted "normal" at least as badly as I did.

On our way to the museum, we passed what I assumed was an old, abandoned airstrip. Suddenly, I was overcome with the urgent need to pray. It wasn't simply something I wanted to do; it was something I had to do right then and there. "Stop the van," I pleaded. "Stop the van."

Michael refused; he could clearly see where things were headed. He must have flashed back immediately to that terrible night in front of our pastor's home. Refusal, I think, was his last ditch attempt to avert a crisis.

It didn't work. When he wouldn't stop, I opened the door of the van and jumped out. We weren't going very fast, so I was not injured. I immediately began walking toward the airstrip; it seemed to beckon me. As I got there, I began to repeat, *"In the name of Jesus, I rebuke you. In the name of Jesus, I rebuke you,"* over and over again. I walked the entire length of the airstrip chanting my prayer. I didn't know why I was doing this or who I was addressing, but it answered a need I felt deep in my soul.

At one point, I remember looking back and seeing my husband. He was following me, carrying our son. After a moment, it registered that he was calling my name; he was asking me to stop. But I couldn't; that was literally beyond my power.

I looked back again and saw that my husband had stopped to speak to someone. That barely registered in the moment, but it turns out the airstrip was not abandoned. Planes still took off and landed there. I was creating a hazard and the police had come to investigate.

By this time, I had come to the end of the airstrip and I started walking down the road that ran beside it, still praying. Slowly it dawned on me that a police car was following me very slowly. After a few minutes, an officer got out of the car and ran to catch up with me. I didn't mind at all; I was not afraid.

I let the officer convince me that it was okay for him to take me some place safe. I don't think I understood exactly what was happening. I believed I was on a mission to eliminate a past evil; maybe I thought his coming was part of the plan. He would take me where I needed to go. Where exactly didn't matter much to me at that point; I would confront the evil wherever I found it. My prayers had placed me under God's protection and I was at peace.

The officers took me to an old building. One went inside while the driver and I waited in the car. I remember that the officer in the car with me asked me what was happening.

For some reason I said, "My husband and I had an argument." I indicated that it was a family matter I would not discuss. Inside the building, through the doorway, I could see my husband and son. Michael looked shaken.

The second officer did not return and, after a time, the officer with me started the car and told me that he was taking me to the safe place I'd been promised. That turned out to be a hospital emergency room. As we sat there, waiting to talk to a doctor, I heard a familiar song, sung by a Christian artist. Though the sound system in the emergency room was less than ideal, it brought me considerable comfort.

By the time I got to talk to the health care workers, some of my certainty had drained away and I was dead tired. But I was able to tell them how I was feeling—though I omitted the fact that I had spent two entirely sleepless nights. Why I did this, I don't know, but what I told them was enough that they decided to admit me, particularly when I explained that I had been given a mission to help someone. And I was willing to be admitted. I would, I thought, be safe there and maybe I would meet the person I was directed to help.

They treated me kindly, more kindly that I had been treated at any hospital in the past. I believe that part of the reason for this was that the officer who had caught up with me on the road by the airstrip was a police chaplain. I think he understood what I was experiencing much better than anyone else would have. Clearly I was ill, but I was also undergoing a significant spiritual experience. Sometimes there is no neat separation between these two states.

Another hospital confinement was devastating. I had come so far in recovery and this setback had come suddenly at a time when I was doing particularly well. What had caused my relapse? Had it been the spiritual pressures I'd been subject to at the campground, those two days of gradually increasing awareness before the more bizarre occurrences began? Or was it simply a change in location and a couple nights of sleeplessness? To the hospital staff, the spiritual experiences I described were nothing more than symptoms of my illness, and they immediately placed me on anti-psychotic medication. I could not dismiss my experiences so easily, however, and even with the anti-psychotic medication, they did not completely subside. At night, I was still hyper aware and unable to sleep. It seemed to me that I felt the presence of every evil or tragic thing that had happened at the hospital or the surrounding town. Now I didn't hear anyone speak directly to me, and I did not see anything that was not physically present, but the enveloping fog of evil was nearly as oppressive as it had been at the campsite. To the hospital staff, the only solution was more medication. They seemed to consider no other option.

Even in my confused state, I could see that there was a link between my relapse and what was happening to me spiritually, but I was—and still am—convinced that the link was much more complex than that. I think it would have helped me greatly to speak, at length, with a spiritually knowledgeable pastor, priest, or minister. I needed to talk to someone whose frame of reference at least allowed the possibility that something more was occurring—someone who could speak to my soul. Had I had this opportunity at the onset of my relapse, I think I would not have become as suspicious and paranoid as I did in the hospital.

This is not to say, though, that I had no grounds for suspicion. One evening while I was in the hospital, I began to have difficulty speaking during one of the group meetings. I could not seem to think clearly and something seemed to be stopping my throat from working properly. I managed to get through the night without too much discomfort, but by the next morning I could not speak at all.

Fortunately, my husband came to see me early that morning. When he came into the visiting room, I couldn't speak to greet him, and soon afterwards, I began drooling from my mouth. I couldn't control it and it wouldn't stop. That was enough for Michael to guess what was going on. From previous experience, he knew enough to ask one of the nurses, "Did my wife receive the medicine that prevents the side effects of the anti-psychotic medication?" Almost immediately afterwards, the nurse gave me a shot. Soon I could swallow normally, and soon after that I regained the ability to speak. Michael had seen immediately what the nurses had missed for hours. That was not reassuring.

And, whatever else I was going through, I was an experienced businesswoman who had spent years working in the health care industry. I was familiar with standard practices, especially those procedures a professional should follow to prevent contamination or contagion. So when the nurse who was preparing to take my blood laid the needle she planned to use on the ground, I was shocked by her carelessness. "You will not take my blood," I said, insisting that she follow the proper procedures for handling sterile equipment.

My "attitude" didn't endear me to the staff. In fact, it earned me a reputation as a "difficult" patient. The fact that I began to share my procedural knowledge with other patients didn't help that much either, but I had learned through years of bitter experience that psychiatric hospitals are not like other hospitals. Psychiatric hospitals routinely treat patients like prisoners who don't know how to care for themselves. You would think individuals working in a psychiatric hospital would be the people most likely to understand that mental illness does not necessarily imply stupidity or diminished capacity; the first to understand that people with mental illness can be partners in their own treatment. Yet, in my experience, this simply isn't the case. Typically doctors and mental health workers spend little time with patients. They are usually given very little information about new patients to begin with, and they then make care decisions after very cursory exams that often last no more than minutes. Only rarely are patients given full physical and mental evaluations; a patient's spiritual condition is almost always left out completely.

Worse, patients are almost never informed about their treatment. The doctors are remote figures who drop by very occasionally and the health workers upon whom they depend for routine treatment don't bother to explain what they are doing and why. Given these conditions, it isn't really surprising that a patient's paranoia will often intensify while he or she is confined.

Not long before I was to be discharged, I asked a nurse if I could speak with my case manager or doctor. "They are not available, "she replied. "They are meeting to review patient cases."

I was furious. Months, even years, of frustration came to a head at that moment. I was tired of being treated like a child. No, actually it was worse than that; adults usually try to tailor their explanations to a child's developmental level. I was being left out entirely, as I had been from the beginning of my illness. As calmly as I could, I asked, "If they are talking about my case, why wasn't I invited to attend?"

The nurse had no answer; you would have thought I was asking for a seat on the next space shuttle. It was clear to me that I would have to push the issue. I calmly and firmly demanded to see the doctor or caseworker immediately.

When that was denied, I had finally had enough. From the nurses' station I could see the staff meeting room. The mini-blinds on the window were raised where they all were. I walked up, banged on the window, and demanded they let me in. That was a mistake, of course. No one made any attempt to talk to me or calm me down. Instead, I was forced into a hospital room, strapped to a bed, and given a shot. That might have been standard hospital procedure, but it terrified me. I was sure they were going to kill me. I remember saying, "You will be forgiven," before I lost consciousness.

I remember nothing more until a hospital staff member came into the room to release the straps. I realized my husband and family were there as well, and relief washed over me. I had lived. I was even hungry, something I had not felt in days. Then my husband gave me a card; that day was our eleventh anniversary. The card was beautiful, but it was all I could do not to weep. I had wanted our anniversary to be perfect and, instead, we were here. That must be my fault, I thought; I had been stable for more than a year, but that apparently was not enough.

They told me that the goal was to stabilize me enough so that I could make the drive home. Then, I would resume care with my regular psychiatric doctor—the woman who had initially stabilized me and who had changed the direction of my recovery. Of course, I wanted to go home, and I wanted to leave Asheville. I still thought this strange, bizarre place was responsible for at least some of what had happened to me. So I was willing to ignore what seemed to me to be the elephant in the room. How could I become stable when I did not know what was causing me to become unstable? I decided not to ask questions and just go along with the program as best I could.

Now, I would say, "Question, question, question! Doctors are human, too. They make mistakes, and they sometimes omit important information. Ask until you get the answers you need; the answers you deserve."

Every human being is unique, but the standard medical system is based on groups and classes. Up to a point, of course, this is useful; common factors among groups and classes often provide valuable information for the diagnosis and treatment of illnesses. The problem is that all too often it is a limited approach. A patient becomes no more than an illness and everything else about the person is dismissed. In this model it doesn't matter that a patient with a broken leg is also a professional violinist. Or that he or she is a practicing Christian, or Jew, or Hindu for that matter. None of these things fit into the paradigm of classes and groups. By now I knew that my illness had affected all of me—body, mind, and spirit. The doctors in North Carolina, like most of the other health care professionals I had met during my years of treatment, seemed ill prepared to treat me as a whole, unique human being. Like most people in our culture, I had been brought up not to question a doctor's authority and it took me a long time to get past that. Now I think that asking more questions and asking until I got serious, well-thought-out answers might have spared me years of limited treatment.

Many of the answers I needed had been there all along. It turns out that spiritual experiences like mine are actually typical of postpartum psychosis. Most women have visions or hear voices. Every doctor or counselor with experience in postpartum psychosis had to have known this. Why was I in treatment for more than three years before a counselor finally told me? And why, if the phenomenon is so common, does there seem to be no standard procedure for helping a woman deal with the spiritual ramifications of her illness?

Five days after we had arrived in Asheville, we left for home. Michael's parents had driven to North Carolina from Pennsylvania as soon as he called to tell them I had been admitted to the hospital, and my mother-in-law decided to drive back to Florida with us so she could help. Her presence was a huge blessing. The medication I was on made it impossible for me to drive, so she took turns with Michael driving us home. And she gave him the emotional support he badly needed. My relapse had been as devastating for him as it had been for me.

As soon as I got home, I made an appointment to see my doctor. The first thing she asked me about was the medication I was taking. It turned out the dosages were much too high—presumably because the doctor in North Carolina had increased them to control my experiences— and she adjusted them immediately. Michael and I described to her what had happened during our trip and how concerned we were that I had relapsed without warning. She worked with me, adjusting my medications as needed until I became stable again. This time, however, she decided not to take me off medication completely once I had stabilized. I would continue to take one of the medications to help me remain stable. I still did not know why I had relapsed in the first place or why I would continue to need medication, but of course I took it anyway. I wanted to be well.

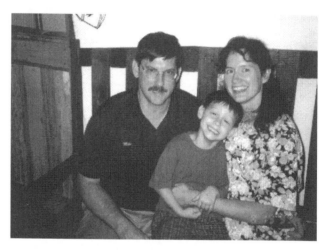

One month after trip to North Carolina in 1999.

By August 1999, one month after our trip to North Carolina, I was stable and doing well. The rash on my ankle still had not gone away though, so I was referred to a dermatologist. He gave me another cream to try, but he also ordered a blood glucose test. He told me that skin rashes can be a symptom of diabetes. He wanted to eliminate that possibility, and in fact, the test came back normal. After another few weeks, the rash itself faded. We never did figure out what had caused it.

What I didn't know then was that blood sugar levels can also be a factor in psychosis. Was that a factor in what had happened to me in North Carolina? It is true that I lost my appetite during that period and ate nothing for a period of days, but I can only speculate now. By the time I had the glucose test, well after I had already stabilized again, the results would not have reflected my condition prior to the trip.

Much later I learned that anti-psychotic medications can affect blood sugar levels as well. In addition, my understanding is that problems either with blood sugar levels or thyroid function can mimic depression and anxiety as well as psychosis. Every woman who suffers from any symptoms of mental illness related to childbearing—and certainly everyone who suffers from psychosis—should test their blood sugar and thyroid function regularly.

Michael and I also went back to our marriage and family counselor. At his request, we asked the hospital in North Carolina to fax the records of my stay there to him. By the time we saw him for the first time since our return, he had already received them. As he ushered us into his office, he said, "I nearly fell out of bed when I read the hospital's notes. I'd just come down off a hiking trip in the mountains and was less than ten miles away that night." So close, yet so far; this is the one man with whom I was able to discuss my spirituality. It might have made an incredible difference had I been able to see him while I was hospitalized. Still, I told him in detail what I had experienced in Asheville, and that conversation added another level to our discussions.

We started to talk about some of the spiritual aspects of my illness we had not yet explored.

Of course, standard medical treatment played an enormous role in my recovery, and I am grateful to all of the doctors and health care professionals who treated me. I believe that medicine, therapy, and support are essential to recovery, but they are not all that is needed. Failure to address the spiritual aspects of an illness can delay or even prevent recovery. My body and mind were healing nicely, but my spirit was still wounded. My bizarre trip to North Carolina, painful and tortuous as it was, helped me begin the process of spiritual healing.

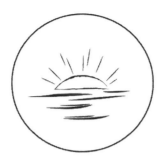

Chapter 9

The Big Move

In February 2000 the recovery-changing female doctor I had been seeing for the last three years moved to a different state, and I began to look for a new doctor. I wanted to find someone with whom I could develop the kind of relationship I had enjoyed with her. She had been the first doctor to speak *with me* rather than *to me* about my treatment, and I was sure that was one of the primary reasons for the success we gained. I also wanted my new doctor to be an expert in women's health.

And I was looking for one other quality. In the two years since my initial recovery, I had met a couple of other women whose experiences after childbearing had been similar to mine. I had been able to help provide them with the kind of emotional support that is crucial to recovery. One of them, a woman who suffered from postpartum depression (PPD), said to me one day, "You are the only person I can talk to about this; the only person who can understand how I feel." I knew exactly what she meant; I remembered all too well the terrible isolation I had felt. Talking to her that day clarified something for me that had been slowly building. I wanted to do more of this work. And I wanted to find a doctor who would understand this and support my decision.

After a time, I thought I had found her. I made an appointment to see a doctor with an extensive background in women's health issues. Even better, my insurance company confirmed that they would cover her treatments. I was looking forward to seeing her.

That's when doors began to close all around me. The first closure came two weeks before my scheduled appointment with my new doctor. Her office called to say that she too was moving out of state and that, since this was the case, she thought it best not to take on new patients.

I was disappointed, but not too concerned. I still had plenty of medication and my previous doctor had given me her new home number. I could always reach her in the event of an emergency, but I was doing well enough now that a crisis seemed unlikely. Also, Michael and I were still seeing our marriage and family counselor. Sessions with him seemed to help more than anything else at this point.

Then a second door closed. My husband had trained for a new position at work and had been promised a promotion. Right before he was scheduled to start his new job, he was informed that he would receive no increase to his current salary. Understandably, he was very upset. Besides the fact that an increase would have reflected the extra work he had put in and his increased value to the company, we had been counting on the money. Our son was now 4 years old and would be starting school soon. That would mean new expenses, and we had counted on his increased salary to meet them.

That led to the closing of the third door. At the time we lived there, the schools in our area were over-crowded and had discipline problems. Something needed to be done to improve the situation and citizens had put considerable pressure on the county government to, among other things, tie future growth to school capacity. When the county officials voted not to do this, I began to consider moving. A private school would be beyond our means and the public school system was now not likely to improve. Leaving the area seemed the best option to me.

"What are the chances of moving to a new area?" I asked my husband.

At first, he was reluctant to even consider the idea, but we brought the matter up the next time we saw our marriage counselor. It was a painful discussion, but one that we needed to have. It gave Michael the opportunity to talk about some of what he'd been through during my illness. He had been affected by it almost as profoundly as I had, but as husband, father, and primary provider he had felt he needed to be strong and contain his own emotions. Now he could talk about how hard the last few years had been for him and how concerned he was about future problems. He had been frustrated by his job for a long time, but he hesitated to make any changes for fear it would jeopardize the stability we'd worked so hard to maintain. He felt stuck at work, but taking any risk seemed selfish and irresponsible to him. He thought people would judge him pretty harshly if he took any risks for the sake of his own happiness.

The counselor encouraged Michael to consider making some changes and to let his own needs be part of the equation. "As long as you know you're right with God," he said, "it should not matter what anyone else thinks."

Talking to the counselor and expressing some of his own thoughts and fears helped Michael see the possibilities of a move. He grew much more receptive to the idea. Our son was much harder to convince. When his father and I told him that we might move, he immediately came back with, "I don't want to leave my friends." That crystallized for us the importance of moving relatively soon. We wanted to give him plenty of time to make new friends before he started school.

Moving isn't a big deal to many people, but for us it was a major change. Both Michael and I had spent our entire childhoods in one town. We had both lived in one house until we left home as adults. He had worked at the same job for the last ten years, and we had lived in our house for nine years. We weren't the kind of people who made changes at the drop of a hat. In addition, we were close to much of my family. My father, sisters, and brother all lived about an hour from us. But once we finally made the decision to go, things seemed to fall into place quickly for us.

Our first step was to research the possibilities and determine the best location for us. We began with a list of the things that were most important. We knew, for example, that we wanted to stay in the same state. Not only did that keep us relatively close to my family, we liked the fact that we paid no state income tax. Second, since my husband worked in the aviation industry, our new home would have to be located in an area in which he could find a job. Finally, we wanted to live in a location that had an excellent public school system. The list helped us narrow down our choices to three top locations. We settled in for what we were sure was going to be the hard part—locating job possibilities for Michael in our selected areas and arranging for interviews.

It actually didn't take long at all. One afternoon Michael called. He sounded excited and optimistic as he said, "I'm eligible to transfer to a good job in my company. It's located in the area we selected as our first choice." It had been less than a month since we decided to move.

I was thrilled and Michael immediately applied. He was selected for an interview and offered the job soon after he went through the interview. Now we had to move quickly. We contacted a realtor to put the house on the market as soon as possible. With the work Michael had done over the years, it didn't take much to get the house ready, and it sold in a week to a member of our church. We loved our house while we lived there and were delighted that it would go to a family we knew.

Throughout this period I had done well. My health was good and the impending change had neither made me particularly anxious nor disrupted my sleep patterns. About a month before our move, however, I came down with a cold that quickly turned into bronchitis. The coughing kept me awake at night and my sleep began to suffer. To make matters worse, my son came down with scarlet fever. With proper medicine, rest, and care he recovered quickly, but his illness took a toll on me. My emotions were always going to be fragile where his health was concerned, and caring for him further eroded my sleep patterns.

These were warning signs I had to take seriously, so I consulted my primary care physician who prescribed a sleeping pill. The medication helped restore my sleep patterns and by about two weeks before our scheduled move I was sleeping normally. The doctor did more than this however; she referred me to a psychiatrist who could prescribe more of the medication I had been taking since our trip to North Carolina. I followed the recommendation and saw her. She renewed the prescriptions and recommended that, once I got to our new location, I should discuss other medicine options with my new doctor. As I was leaving, she followed all this up with, "Be sure to take the medicine during the move and transition."

I agreed, of course, but I was also frustrated by what amounted to a cryptic warning. After all, I had been taking the same medication for about a year. Why would I suddenly stop? Why was there a particular emphasis on taking it during the move? Was my body now so sensitive to any kind of stress—positive or negative—that instability was a permanent danger? The doctor did not explain herself; I was used to this by now, but that made it no less frustrating.

It would be some time before I learned that the particular kind of stress makes a difference. Major life changes, for example, are known to trigger symptoms of anxiety and depression, especially when they occur in pregnancy or in the postpartum period. There are ways to manage this stress, including therapy and practical support and, if necessary, appropriate medication. So, obviously, in my situation the doctor was right to emphasize that I take the medication. However, more specific information about the risks I faced, and what I could do to lessen them, would have been extremely helpful. Fortunately for us, both Michael and I come from close families from whom this kind of support is second nature. We had the support we needed and avoided any crises. Many families are not as fortunate, and all too many women suffer from relapses they might have avoided had they had the appropriate information to manage their risks.

Twelve days before our scheduled move, my niece was to be married in Pennsylvania. Michael knew how much I wanted to be there, so he volunteered to say home and finish the packing while my son and I traveled north for the wedding. We made the trip without incident and I enjoyed the wedding and the family gathering that followed. Then I came home to help Michael with the final arrangements for the move. Michael's mother, my son's "Nanny," came down from Pennsylvania to help us with the move.

Moving day dawned bright and clear. The movers loaded some of our belongings into a rented trailer, while Michael hitched our camper to the van. It would be our home while we looked for a new house. Then, Michael climbed into the trailer, while Nanny, my son, and I piled into the van for the 11-hour trip to our new hometown. While I drove, Nanny kept my son occupied with toys, games, and stories. The miles flew by and I was incredibly grateful for the presence of another adult.

If anything, my gratitude increased over the next few weeks. While Michael and I shopped for a new house, my mother-in-law took care of our son. This made our search much easier and in about two weeks we found the perfect house. It was lovely, affordable, and located in a neighborhood with great schools. It satisfied even our toughest critic. "I never want to go back to our old house," was our son's verdict when he saw it. I felt a deep sense of peace; the ease of our move had shown me that we were right where God wanted us to be.

I had another blessing as well. Before I left our old home, I had tried to arrange a job transfer with the national retail store that employed me part-time. Due to a hiring freeze, however, they had been unable to accommodate my request. That disappointment faded when we reached our new town, much smaller than the one we had left, and I realized that I would have had a 45-minute commute to the closest store. Since full-time daycare was not in our budget, I got the unexpected gift of caring for my son full-time. I had lost so much time with him during the worst of my illness and his school years were fast approaching. I decided to cherish the time.

Once we settled in, finding new doctors and a counselor became my priority. I quickly found a primary care doctor for our entire family who had a holistic view of patient care. Finding a new counselor took a while longer. My husband was reluctant at first; he believed we no longer needed counseling. I, on the other hand, was committed to continuing; appropriate counseling had been vital to overcoming the effects of my illness on our marriage. Just as regular oil changes keep a car running for the life of the engine, I believe that counseling can help keep a marriage running for life. Michael was open to persuasion, and I was able to find a new counselor whose spiritual values were in alignment with our own.

I was also able to locate a female psychiatrist with some experience with postpartum-related mental illness. I arranged to meet with her and we hit it off immediately. After all I had been through I was now very particular about my doctor. I wanted to be sure I could trust the person in whose hands I was putting my life and health, and I now knew how to ask much better questions to be sure I had found her. When my hair started falling out, much more than the usual amount I noticed on my brush, I felt comfortable talking to her about this. She told me that my current medication could cause this, and recommended a mineral pill to help with this. It worked and cemented out relationship that much more.

Finding medical care I could trust brought me great peace of mind. I don't think there was a single moment of insight or anything like a brilliant flash; it just slowly dawned on me that I now had everything I had wanted when I looked forward to my son's birth. He was healthy and thriving. I was healthy and happy and my marriage to Michael was strong and loving. He was happier in his new job, and best of all, I was the healthy, happy, full-time mother I had dreamed of being. I thought my cup of joy had run over.

I didn't know that a whole new door would shortly open for me.

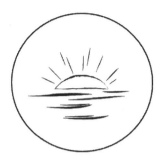

Chapter 10

Putting the Pieces Together

I first spoke with Jane Honikman, the founder of Post-partum Support International (PSI), in June of 2000. By then we had happily settled into our new home and I had time again to pursue my ambition to help other women going through the trauma of mental illness related to childbearing. I had volunteered at the crisis pregnancy center, but though I had enjoyed it and felt I made a contribution, I had primarily done administrative work. Now I wanted to do more. In the year or so before we moved, I'd met and supported several women dealing with emotional illnesses related to childbearing. These experiences had been personal and ad-hoc, but they confirmed an idea that had grown out of the isolation of my own illness. I could make an enormous difference because I had been where they were. Most of the people around them were either entirely unaware of postpartum mental illnesses or aware of them only through sensationalized media accounts of tragedies. The isolating veil of stigma and ignorance was—and sometimes still is—nearly as traumatizing as the illness itself.

PSI is a non-profit organization whose mission is to raise awareness of health issues related to childbearing, and to work for prevention and treatment of these illnesses. I had actually been a member of the organization for a while; that is, I had been on their mailing list and received their information. I had never actually spoken with anyone from the organization.

So when I called PSI to update my mailing address information, I expected a brief, rather routine conversation. Instead, the courteous woman who answered the phone identified herself as Jane Honikman, the organization's founder.

We had a wonderful, enlightening conversation. This was the first time I had spoken with someone experienced in the kind of work I wanted to do. Keep in mind that this was 2000, and the internet was far more limited than it is now. The resources available today were little more than ambitious dreams then. It would take several more years of work by many dedicated people before they came into being. In meeting Jane I thought I had struck gold. It was thrilling and emotional for me. I remember telling her, "If I can help just one person, it would all be worth it." I gave her my new mailing address, of course, but I also told her that I would love to become more involved with PSI. I wanted to know how to get started.

Jane promised to help and she followed up on that promise. She put me in touch with two PSI volunteer coordinators who lived in my state, and through them I began to learn about the vast worldwide need for information and support in the area of mental health issues related to childbearing. I also learned a great deal about these illnesses that I had never known before, despite the years I had been in treatment for postpartum psychosis. It was now time to go back and look at my own story through the lens of this new knowledge. This was no stroll down memory lane. I was learning to identify the risk factors in my own case and link them to risk factors common to women worldwide. The problems I had getting adequate and informed care were also part of a far larger pattern. It was as if I started at the center of a labyrinth and walked outward to see where all the paths led and how they all fit together.

So why did I come down with postpartum psychosis? I don't have all the answers, and I don't think anyone does yet. Though postpartum psychosis was first recognized as a disorder in 1850, insight into its causes has come about slowly. Even the exact number of women in the United States who suffer from it is still unknown, since it is frequently misdiagnosed as postpartum depression—a separate, but related, illness.

However, we now have much better information about known risk factors that can alert women and their families to potential problems, and help manage them during pregnancy and after a child's birth. Among the problems that surround the treatment of psychosis in general, and post-partum psychosis in particular, are ignorance, stigma, and the shame attached to these diseases. It is estimated that fewer than 20 percent of women who suffer from postpartum psychosis ever discuss their fears with their health care provider. This means, of course, that they tend to receive appropriate treatment only if and when their symptoms become obvious to others. Even then, those who do receive treatment are often misdiagnosed.

Foreknowledge of any risks, and a greater understanding of mental illness related to childbearing in general, can eliminate a tremendous amount of needless suffering. In fact, women who receive the appropriate treatment for postpartum psychosis generally respond very well to it. Without treatment the results can be tragic.

For most of my childhood I was raised in a single-parent family. My father left us when I was 4 years old, leaving my mother solely responsible for eight children. As was common at the time, she had not worked outside the home for 22 years. Keeping us fed and clothed was a struggle for her, and I grew up determined never to find myself in that position. Evidence suggests that women who suffer childhood traumas, such as the loss of a parent through death or divorce, may have a somewhat higher risk for mental illnesses related to childbearing. By itself, this is hardly a determining factor, but it is one that should be considered in a realistic assessment of any woman's risk.

By the time I entered high school, I had decided I would never marry. That resolution lasted until I met Michael during my sophomore year. We dated for seven years before we married. At first we were not sure whether we wanted to have children together, and since I was still in college anyway, waiting to start a family made sense to us. Besides, I was still determined to have an independent career. No matter how strong my marriage was—and it was strong and loving—I was determined that what happened to my mother would never happen to me. It took a long time, and a lot of trust, before I could let that go.

I launched my career and enjoyed it, but slowly, over time I began to realize that I did want a child. The desire grew, and by the time Michael and I celebrated our fifth wedding anniversary, I knew I was ready to become a mother. Michael was ready for parenthood as well.

I followed the doctor's advice and waited until I had been off birth control pills for three months before I began to try to get pregnant. Once we began to try, we found it wasn't as easy as we had hoped it would be. Months went by, and I began to get concerned. I wondered if I was suffering from the long-term effects of the birth control pills I had been taking. But I knew plenty of women who had been on the pill for a long time, and who still had no difficulty getting pregnant when they decided the time was right. I began to fear I might have more serious fertility problems. The year that passed before I became pregnant seemed to drag on for an eternity.

Finally we got the news we'd been waiting for; Michael and I were elated. I was about six weeks pregnant when we told our families and friends that we were expecting a child. My in-laws were especially excited; our child would be their first grandchild. Two weeks later, I miscarried.

It was late afternoon, and a coworker and I paused to chat in the parking lot before we left for the evening. Suddenly, I felt as if my period had begun. Since that was something that shouldn't have been happening, I quickly said my goodbyes and got into my car. Discretely as I could, I checked my underwear. It was true; I was definitely bleeding. Frantic with concern, I drove to the emergency room as quickly as I could. Thank goodness it wasn't far away.

As soon as I entered the building, I told the reception nurse that I was pregnant and bleeding. She made sure I saw a doctor as soon as possible. He was initially reassuring. "Sometimes pregnant women can bleed without ill effect," he said. That calmed my fears a bit, but as soon as I was taken to an emergency room bed, I called my husband. "I'm bleeding," I said.

He was stunned. "I'll be there right away," he promised. Since I had the car, he had to ask a neighbor to drive him, but he made it to the hospital in record time. He was there with me when the ultrasound was administered. He was there when the doctor came back to tell me the results. The ultrasound had shown an empty fetal sac. "I'm so sorry," he said. "You have had a missed abortion." That's the term they use when a baby dies or fails to grow. It sounded chillingly clinical and we knew it was final. Our child would never be born. We held each other and cried. What I wouldn't know for years was that having had a previous miscarriage put me at greater risk for postpartum mental illness.

My regular doctor was out of town that day, so I was assigned a different doctor for the follow-up care I would need. I would have to have a surgical procedure called a dilation and curettage (D&C). The doctor would essentially scrape my womb to ensure that no dead tissue remained. Since dead tissue can pose a serious health risk, the surgery would happen as soon as the doctor they'd assigned could get to the hospital. Michael went back to the house to pick up a few things I would need for the hospital say.

While I was waiting for him to get back, the doctor arrived. He described to me exactly what he was going to do. I asked it if would be possible to wait until Michael got back before he began the surgery. "I'm sorry," he replied, "Waiting is not an option." By now I understood the risks, but I was already nervous about having an unfamiliar doctor perform the surgery. Knowing that Michael would not be there when I went under anesthesia made my fear that much greater. But there didn't seem to be any other reasonable choice.

The worst pain I experienced during the miscarriage or the treatment that followed was the catheter the hospital staff inserted into my bladder prior to the surgery. Every time I moved, pain would shoot up my groin. That was the one thing that made me glad the surgery would happen quickly; it would be removed during the procedure.

When I awoke in the recovery room a nurse told me the surgery had gone well. I was glad to hear it. I was even happier to see that Michael was waiting for me when they took me from the recovery room. I would have to stay in the hospital until I could urinate without a catheter. I remember making up my mind that would happen very quickly. I was over the entire concept of catheters.

My body healed very quickly from the miscarriage, but my spirit had taken a beating and recovered much more slowly. I grieved my tiny, unborn child as I would have grieved the death of anyone I loved. I learned that this was not unusual; most women do experience grief after such an event. I began to hear stories from women all around me who had gone through miscarriages. My mother and one of my sisters each had one. One of my neighbors had experienced two miscarriages. When I went to my regular doctor for follow-up care, she said, "I understand. I miscarried too."

She explained to me that miscarriages are very common. Having already heard so many stories in such a short a time, I could easily believe her. She stunned me, however, when she added, "The usual process is to start looking for a cause or specific problem once a woman has miscarried at least three times." I couldn't imagine going through this loss and sadness two more times. Once had been more than enough.

As C. S. Lewis told us, grief is not a state but a process. This was the first real grief I had suffered in my life, and I discovered that you don't go through it from beginning to end in a logical, orderly fashion and then get done with it. It has laws of its own. One day you think you're doing better, then the next your pain is as fresh as it was in the beginning. And it's something you go through alone; no two people grieve in the same way. My husband seemed to recover more quickly than I did. Maybe it's because my pregnancy ended so early. I had begun to feel the physical changes pregnancy causes, even though no one else could see them yet. Michael, my family, and friends did their best to support me through the grief that followed my miscarriage, but I think the baby was real to me in a way that wasn't yet possible for them. There was no record of my child's brief existence or death, and neither my husband nor I were offered grief counseling. I now think that counseling after a miscarriage should be routinely offered to women and their families—no matter how early or far along in the pregnancy it occurs. In addition to supporting them through the grief and loss, it can help women answer the kind of questions that haunted me for weeks afterwards: Why did this happen? Did I do something wrong?

Counseling would be valuable for one other reason as well: A previous miscarriage is a significant risk factor for mental illness related to childbearing. My doctor advised me to wait at least three months before I tried to get pregnant again, but I don't remember any discussion of other risk factors. Knowing the risks of mental illness related to childbearing can help women make informed decisions about if and when to get pregnant again, enabling them to work with their health care providers to manage this risk.

The heartache of my miscarriage only intensified our desire to become parents as soon as we could. We agreed to start trying again as soon as the recommended three months had passed. It took a little longer than we had hoped, but just about a year after my miscarriage I found out that I was pregnant for the second time. Of course I was delighted, but this time my emotions were guarded. I had learned that most miscarriages occur within the first 12 weeks of pregnancy. I tried to hold back my emotions; I didn't think I could go through the heartbreak of having my joy so cruelly shattered again. For the first few weeks Michael and I told no one. We waited.

It seemed to me like I was holding my breath for the entire time, but finally the fateful deadline passed. I remember the joy of hearing my baby's heartbeat for the first time— one week short of the anniversary of my miscarriage. I had an ultrasound a short time later and that confirmed that the baby was healthy.

Now I could enjoy my pregnancy. We told our family and friends that I was pregnant and began to plan for the new arrival. My life seemed to go exceptionally well during this period; my pregnancy was easy and I felt well for almost all of it. I ate well and continued to exercise until my due date was very close. In addition, I received a long sought-after promotion at work. I became a supervisor, something I had worked hard to achieve. I loved my job, and when I left for maternity leave I still planned to return in 12 weeks. I didn't know then that career women often have a harder time adjusting to motherhood. Is this a risk factor for postpartum psychosis and depression, or is it just a feature of modern life? The evidence is still out on that question.

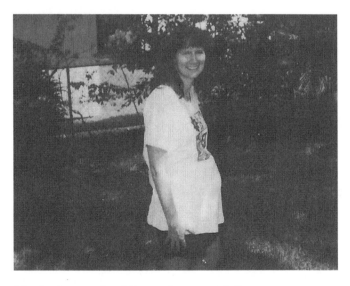

Me during my healthy and uneventful pregnancy

I went into labor on a Wednesday evening, about ten days before my due date. I'd had an instinct that my time was approaching. It was nothing specific—no labor pains or other symptoms—just the growing certainty that I should finish writing the proposal I was currently working on. I needed to have it done before I left for maternity leave, and now I was sure this would be my last opportunity. I stayed late at work to finish it and put the completed proposal on my boss's desk as I left for home. I ate dinner, wrote checks to pay a few bills, and went to bed around 11:00 pm.

I woke suddenly later that night. I looked at the bedside clock and saw that it was 1:20 a.m. I felt a painful cramping in my abdomen. I lay in bed for a while, waiting to see what was happening, trying to decide if I should wake Michael. The cramps continued, but there was a long period between each one. I was pretty sure my labor was beginning.

It was now Thursday morning, but not just any Thursday. It was Thanksgiving Day, and we were expecting my sister, Lynette, and her family for dinner. It was apparent that my son did not care about any of this. He was ready to come into the world and everything else would just have to give way. As soon as we decently could, we called Lynette to tell her our plans were precarious. As you might imagine, she didn't mind; she wanted to come and be with us in case my labor progressed quickly. She offered to take much of the cooking off my hands to make the day as easy as possible, and I wanted them to be there with me.

By mid-morning my cramps were ten minutes apart and quite strong. Michael thought it was time to go to the hospital. I wasn't so sure. I still thought I was in the early stages of labor, and I had a house full of guests coming. Still,

I agreed to go, thinking they would almost certainly examine me and then send me back home for a while

Unfortunately, that's not the way it happened; I was admitted immediately. Now I think that was not the best decision. Being home with my family for the next few hours would have helped me relax, and I probably would have been able to eat at least some of our Thanksgiving dinner. I hadn't eaten since the night before when I was admitted, and I wouldn't have the opportunity to eat before my delivery was complete.

I had taken childbirth classes to prepare for the birth, but like most first-time mothers I found it difficult to ask questions when things did not go as I had been taught to expect. The first departure was that the nurse asked to place a fetal monitor on me. One of the things I had learned in my childbirth classes is that fetal monitors are often misread. For this reason, the teacher had recommended discouraging their use. In spite of this, I found myself agreeing to the nurse's request. All I asked was that it not remain on long.

What happened to me is not an uncommon experience. When you are in the hospital, possibly in a life-threatening situation, you experience a profound need to trust the doctors and nurses around you. You have placed your life in their hands; it's hard in these circumstances to preserve the critical mindset necessary to ask good questions. But the few minutes that the fetal monitor remained on me caused ramifications that were to determine much of the rest of my delivery.

I was never given an internal pelvic exam. Instead, the monitor alone was used to determine the status of the baby and the stage of my labor. Based on the readings the nurse got, the hospital staff told me that I would have to undergo a cesarean section.

The thought terrified me and it went against everything we had planned for the birth of our child. We wanted as natural a birth as possible with as little intervention as possible. But my main concern was, of course, the health of my son. If he were in danger, of course, I would agree to the procedure, as little as I liked the idea.

The first thing Michael did was to try to call our childbirth teacher for guidance and support. He was never able to reach her; it was Thanksgiving Day after all, and she would not have expected me to go into labor so soon.

In the meantime, the hospital staff started me on a fluid IV in preparation for the cesarean. I was resigned; they had told me the situation was serious and that they needed to go ahead quickly. Soon afterwards though my doctor called. She told me that the nurse had misread the tape from the fetal monitor and that a cesarean would not be necessary after all. "We're going to remove the IV and start over," she said. I felt a tremendous relief; my son was not in danger, and it now looked like I could have the natural delivery I wanted.

Once the IV was removed, my labor pains began to taper off. Soon after, my contractions stopped altogether. My husband and I walked the hallways to help bring labor on again. Since it was Thanksgiving, the building was unusually quiet. There were far fewer hospital personnel there, and fewer patients as well; it was almost eerie to walk through the silence, so we decided to go outside for a while.

When my labor pains returned, they came back with a vengeance. Severe back pain accompanied each contraction and quickly got worse. In the hope of getting a little relief, I tried the whirlpool tub in my hospital room. It didn't help much; when the nurse checked my baby's heart rate soon afterwards, she found that it had increased. That was a significant concern and something had to be done.

I had complete confidence in my doctor, and she was well aware of my goal to have as natural a delivery as possible. She suggested an epidural block, saying "An epidural passes the least amount of anesthesia into the baby's blood stream. It will help relax both you and the baby, which should bring his heart rate down." I was disappointed that I would need an epidural, but my doctor's explanation made me more comfortable with the decision. What troubled me more than that was the fact that despite the intense pain, I was still not far along in the labor process. In addition, once I had the epidural I would be unable to eat and I'd had nothing since the previous evening. Any part of the lovely Thanksgiving dinner I had planned was now out of the question.

A nurse anesthetist gave me the epidural about eight o'clock that evening. I remember him saying "You have a perfect spine for this procedure." I thought that was a slightly odd thing to say as a compliment, but he just meant that he could see my spine easily, which made it much easier to insert the needle.

The epidural began to help immediately and as the pain lessened, I began to focus more on the other aspects of labor. I listened to the rhythm of the baby's heartbeat and was reassured as it began to come down, just as the doctor had promised. But the continual "beep, beep, beep" of the fetal monitor made it difficult to relax and prevented me from getting any sleep. Every time I was close to dropping off, it seemed that the sounds changed and startled me back awake. Now I wish I had asked the nurse to turn the volume off.

By 2:00 a.m. I was exhausted. It had been more than 24 hours since I first woke up with labor pains, and the hours had taken a physical toll. The pushing during the last stages of hard labor lasted more than two hours. My husband was there to encourage me and my doctor helped me stay focused. With each push the baby's head would start to come out, but as soon as I stopped pushing it would go back in. I remember Michael saying, "You can do this! Remember that you don't want a cesarean." But my strength was giving out. Someone gave me oxygen and that seemed to help a little, but I began to think I might die before the baby came. I clearly remember calling out, "Oh my God, help me!" It was the only prayer I was able to make.

My mother, who lived more than 1,100 miles away, and my sister, Lynette, who had been with me in the hospital earlier that evening, both later told me that they woke up suddenly at 4:00 a.m. feeling the need to pray for me. This was almost certainly at the same time I made my frantic prayer. Our prayers were answered. At 4:28 a.m. on Friday morning, the day after Thanksgiving, my beautiful son was born. As his head came out, my vaginal skin began to tear, so the doctor had to make a longer surgical cut (episiotomy) to help me deliver him. She also assisted the delivery with a vacuum extractor.

It was over. My baby was here, and he was whole and perfect. I was deeply grateful and completely exhausted. I felt like a ship that had made it safely to the harbor after an arduous voyage. I only wanted to rest and recover. I thought I was through the hard part. I had no idea what was to follow; no idea at all that a long and difficult delivery puts a mother at greater risk for a mood disorder after the birth of a child.

I quickly learned that I wasn't going to get a chance to recover in the hospital. For one thing, my stay was much too short. In 1995, only a 24-hour hospital stay was required after a vaginal delivery. I thought I was fortunate because my insurance covered a 48-hour stay. I naively thought that meant I would have two nights in the hospital to recover from the physical ordeal of my delivery. Wrong. The clock started at the moment of delivery and time ran out exactly 48 hours later—no matter what time of day that happened to be. In practical terms, that translated to a little over a day.

And that day was packed with activity. Clerical tasks, such as the birth certificate and the newborn pictures, had to be completed, and the nurses and other hospital staff members came into the room continually. The attention was reassuring but I was unable to get any of the sleep I so desperately needed at this point. The one thing that they didn't bring was food. I had to call the nurses' station to ask for a meal. Still, other than hunger and exhaustion, I had no problems I was aware of at that point. In fact, I was exhilarated and joyous.

After more than 24 hours of labor, a fourth-degree episiotomy, and one night's assistance with breastfeeding, I was required to leave the hospital before midnight on Saturday. Of course, we didn't leave that late. I went home about 8:00 p.m. in good spirits and happy, even though I was so sore that I had to sit on a pillow. None of the hospital staff seemed concerned about my condition. That actually comforted me. If they weren't worried, experienced as they were, I figured there was no reason for me to worry either. All I could think about was how much I wanted to go home and sleep.

I'd been home for two days when the "baby blues" hit. My sister, Lynette, had warned me to expect them, so I was more or less prepared. Most mothers experience them. After the birth of her child, a woman's hormonal levels often drop dramatically. She may cry frequently, feel irritable or vulnerable, and sleep poorly. Usually the "blues" last for about two weeks before her body readjusts. My experience was fairly standard.

What was much more unusual is what happened when my breast milk "came in." This happened when my son was about four days old. I went from an A cup to a D cup literally overnight, and the swelling was excruciatingly painful. Since breastfeeding had gone well for me up to this point, I was completely unprepared. I was in agony and the only relief I could get came from placing warm washcloths over my breasts. I don't know what I would have done had my husband not been there to help.

We called the hospital for help, and they advised us to have a breastfeeding specialist come to the house to evaluate me. We would have to pay for this, of course.

When the specialist saw me she said, "Yours is the worst case of breast milk engorgement I've ever seen." Considering that she had worked with breastfeeding mothers for many years, that was quite a statement, though I can't say I was entirely surprised. I couldn't believe the agony I was experiencing could be normal. She recommended an electric breast pump, and I jumped on the suggestion. I would have done just about anything to relieve the pain.

The pump rescued me from further misery and it produced a further benefit. I was producing a plentiful supply of milk, far more than my infant son could actually drink. We were able to freeze some of it. At the time, that simply seemed like a wise thing to do. We never imagined that I would have to be hospitalized twice by the time my son was 3 months old, or that I would have to give up breastfeeding when he was 10 weeks old due to the medication I had been prescribed. Much later, I would learn that stopping breast-feeding suddenly can increase a woman's risk for postpar-tum mental illness.

My sister, Lynette, who lived about an hour away, came to help during the first week after my son was born. She had two children of her own and she prepared us for the onset of the "baby blues." "Be prepared," she said, "for spells of crying that seem to happen for no reason." Once the "blues" started, she helped me get through them. The simple pres-ence of someone who has been there before can be aston-ishingly reassuring, especially when you are feeling over-whelmed and wondering if that feeling will ever go away.

All things considered, my case of the blues was relative-ly mild. After another week my mood stabilized and I be-gan to feel much better. My physical strength had returned as well.

About the same time, my mother came down from Pennsylvania to stay with us for a while. She had planned to come before my son was actually born, but as often happens in real life, their plans didn't dovetail and he arrived about ten days before his scheduled due date. She arrived about a week after his birth and helped enormously. She took over the laundry, cooking, and cleaning while I recovered. And best of all, she provided me with tremendous emotional support. Having given birth to eight children, she was my expert on babies. Like most new mothers, I was learning to take care of my son through "on-the-job" training. Her un-flagging support for those first critical weeks made my life much easier, as did support from my husband, our extend-ed family, and our friends. Members of our church brought meals to our house for the first two weeks.

I am sure that this "wonderful" practical and emotional support is the reason that I did not become ill earlier than I did. Like most fathers in the United States, my husband had to return to work in only a few days. The fact that he worked nights meant he was available to help for only a portion of the day. But once my mother returned home after about five weeks, I took over all the chores she had been helping me perform and concentrated on being a full-time, stay-at-home mom. I loved caring for my son, but I had no idea how isolating staying at home would be. I had met most of the friends I socialized with through work; as a work-ing woman, I simply didn't know many people who stayed home with their children during the day. It's a problem I'd never thought about having, but looking back, I believe it was one of the factors in my own illness. I know that iso-lation is another of the risk factors that increases the likeli-hood of developing a mental illness related to childbearing.

We live in a society that has changed greatly over the last few generations. At one time in our history, mothers of very young children had far greater access to community. Now these women either work or live in suburban communities in which most of their neighbors are away during the day. We haven't yet developed the kinds of social structures that could help parents deal with this change, so individuals have to create their own support. It's a factor all women should consider as they plan for the birth of a child, but a woman who has other risk factors for mental illness related to childbearing will need to pay particular attention to preparing "her" support network.

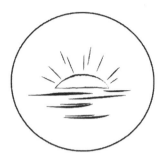

Chapter 11

Advocacy Launched

You've probably heard the saying, "It only takes one person to make a difference." That's true to a certain extent, but when I began to work as an advocate I quickly learned that real, lasting change only occurs when many individuals come together. It requires hard work, detailed knowledge, and perseverance to create hope where there is no hope.

Jane Honikman introduced me to two of the Postpartum Support International (PSI) volunteer coordinators in my state and I began to communicate with them regularly. From our conversations, and from the sources to which they pointed me, I quickly learned more about mental illness related to childbearing than I had ever known. I had taken 12 weeks of childbirth classes prior to my son's birth, and like many expectant mothers, I had read just about everything I could get my hands on. I'd never come across a mention, either in my classes or any of the literature, of mental illness related to childbearing. I had been in treatment for postpartum psychosis for over four years when I began to work with PSI. That, I found, had done shockingly little to remedy my ignorance. By the end of 2000, a substantial body of information was available, but many women still had little or no access to it.

I was determined to change this. I was already spending considerable time talking to the two PSI volunteer coordinators about ways we could expand the much-needed perinatal mental health resources in our state. Now I was ready to take on an official role in the organization. Early in 2001, I became the PSI coordinator for the northwest portion of our state. I would now be responsible for providing emotional, informational, and practical support for families facing mental health challenges related to childbearing. This was similar in many ways to the kind of informal support I'd offered women before we moved. Now I would have a network of resources to help and far more information at my disposal. I was eager to begin.

Soon afterwards, the two other state coordinators and I began initial planning to set up a statewide support network for families. We'd just gotten the project underway when one of the women had to resign as she and her family were moving out of state. That left just two of us to continue. I was fortunate, however, that the remaining coordinator, the coordinator for the southern part of the state, was Ilyene Barsky. She had been one of PSI's first members and was the pioneer in addressing postpartum mental health related issues in our state. Together we made an effective team. Ilyene had tackled the under-addressed issues of perinatal (related to childbearing) mental health, often alone, for years. In fact, we discovered that she lived only an hour and a half away from where I lived when I first became ill. Sadly, I didn't meet her then; it may have been that none of the counselors or doctors I saw at the time knew of her work. A statewide resource network would have solved that problem and Ilyene was delighted to have help bringing it about.

I was the "rookie" still struggling to learn the ropes, and Ilyene was the best possible mentor. The first thing I learned from her is how many layers we would need to peel on this often-overlooked "onion." I had thought the problem was relatively straightforward: Educate women and their families, train the health care providers who treat women, set up a system to provide women and their families with support, and teach self-care. If we managed these things, I thought, we could prevent most mental health issues related to childbearing and cure, at a success rate of 100 percent, those cases that did occur. I decided to take the business-like approach that had worked for me in my career in health care marketing.

I began contacting government officials in my state. I targeted those officials who worked on women's health care issues or for organizations that did. I wanted to contact people with the background and authority to implement change. I quickly ran into a brick wall. I was dealing with a very entrenched bureaucracy that primarily took its direction on women's mental health issues from an equally entrenched medical establishment. For a volunteer organization like PSI, the first, and possibly the most arduous task was getting a "place at the table," that is, acquiring enough of a reputation and enough public support to even be heard.

What we were essentially saying is that the nation has for decades mishandled an important health issue. That's not a message our public servants particularly wanted to hear, and they had less interest in hearing it when the affected constituency lacked the kind of well-heeled lobbying groups that advance careers. Unfortunately, illnesses that only strike women still score pretty low grades on the agendas of most of our leaders. Add in the stigma that surrounds mental health in general, and an illness like postpartum psychosis in particular, and their reluctance intensified.

Then there was the medical establishment. They often don't like hearing that they've taken the wrong path either. There are too many reputations and too much research money tied up in maintaining the status quo. It takes a long time and a concerted effort by many people to even begin change. Seriously addressing the issue of mental health related to childbearing was going to require a shift in the way research into women's health issues was funded and better training of health care providers. Given the nature of the medical establishment, I could see that change was going to have to come from the top.

I dug my heels in and prepared for a long battle. I would spend more than four years "in the trenches" as a volunteer coordinator.

And the good news is that slowly, painfully, we are gaining ground. We have a long way to go, and there are still far too many women who suffer needlessly, but things are beginning to get better. Despite the fact that many of our public servants seem more interested in pursuing their own agendas rather than the public's, there are those who have been willing to support changes in mental health policy.

At the federal level, the first parity law passed was the 1996 Mental Health Parity Act (MHPA). This act mandated that group health plans set the annual and lifetime dollar limits for mental health coverage at no less than the coverage for physical illness. It provided only partial parity since employers with 50 or fewer employees were exempted from the act. Nor were current cases affected. My illness began in early 1996, before the passage of the act, so my health insurance company did not have to offer me the same lifetime maximums for mental illness that they did for physical illness.

Full parity legislation was introduced in Congress during the 2001/2002 session, but failed to pass. It was introduced again in 2003/2004 and 2005/2006, but failed both times. In addition, the law passed in the 1996 was set to expire on December 31, 2007. By the time it did, almost half the states in the country had passed laws to require full parity for mental health coverage. Finally, on October 3, 2008, President George W. Bush signed full mental health parity permanently into law. The legislation still exempts group health care plans that cover fewer than 50 employees, but it was a giant step forward in the long battle to end health insurance discrimination against people seeking treatment for mental illness.

In 2001, supporters introduced H.R. 846, the Melanie Blocker-Stokes Postpartum Depression Research and Care Act into both the House and Senate. This act would have amended the Public Health Service Act to provide research on, and services for, women with postpartum depression and psychosis. The act failed in the 107th congress, and was reintroduced in February 2003. It was referred to committee in each house, but no further action was taken.

The Mom's Opportunity to Access Health, Education, Research, and Support for Postpartum Depression Act, or MOTHERS Act was introduced in Congress in 2006. The act was written to ensure that new mothers and their families are educated about postpartum depression, screened for symptoms, and provided with essential services. In addition, it directed the National Institute of Health to increase funding for research on postpartum depression. The act passed in the House of Representatives in March 2009, and then died in the Senate. The Melanie Blocker-Stokes Postpartum Depression Research and Care Act and the MOTHERS Act were combined and reintroduced into Congress. It passed the Senate as part of the Senate version of the Patient

Protection and Affordable Healthcare Act. It was signed into law as part of that act.

Still, this is only a beginning. We have started to see some major changes at the federal level, and some states have made great progress in educating their citizens and providing access to much-needed care. But there are still too many women who are never diagnosed with mental illnesses related to childbearing, or who are misdiagnosed. This continues to result in avoidable tragedies, the latest of which, at the time of this writing, happened in October 2013 when a woman who "suffered from postpartum depression" was shot and killed by Capitol police after she rammed a White House barricade. Although information about her motives and the situation is sketchy, it is probable that she had limited, if any access to proper support and care. Sadly, we will never know exactly what her experiences were. She will never get to tell us her side of the story.

Proper support and care is an ongoing need. Throughout this period, I considered myself completely recovered from postpartum psychosis, although I knew it had changed me in some ways. I was to find out just how deep those changes ran.

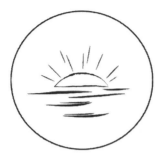

Chapter 12

The Spirit Follows

On the tenth of January 2001, I wrote in my journal, "It's hard to believe only a little more than four years ago, things were so very different for me. I could never have imagined then that I would be where I am now."

My illness and the subsequent period of recovery were the most traumatic, life-changing events of my life. They separated me forever from the person I was before the onset of my illness and, once again, from the person I was during the darkest days of illness. The healthy, happy woman who wrote that diary entry to celebrate a new year was someone I could only dream of becoming in the worst part of my illness.

When you have lived through an experience like my illness, the natural impulse is to look for the meaning in what has happened to you, and to try to create something of value from all of the pain and anguish. Advocacy work had become my way of doing this. The work I did in conjunction with other volunteers at PSI and like-minded people across the country was beginning to make a real difference in women's lives. Because of our efforts, more information about mental health issues related to childbearing was available to women and their health care providers, and fewer women had to go through the experiences I did before they found the care they needed. We still had a great deal to do, but we could look back and see the change for the better that had occurred in only a few years.

This is the "what next" step beyond physical recovery, but it's not a stage that health care providers typically address. Traumatic, life-threatening illnesses are not like simple injuries; they don't end when the bandages are removed or the stitches come out. Your body will never be the same as it was, for example, and you will have to learn all over how to live in and take care of the "new" body you now have. In my own case, I found that none of my health care providers mentioned that I would need a long-term health strategy, much less helped me design one. They were very much focused on my present condition and needs. That was undeniably important, of course, but there seemed to be no transition to managing long-term once the "bandages were off." Nor did there seem to be any way of addressing the emotional and spiritual changes I'd been through in conjunction with my physical recovery.

Many of these issues I had been able to address with our marriage counselor, but there was a real disconnection between these discussions and the rest of the care I received. The standard American medical model still really does not include the non-quantifiable aspects of recovery, and patients are largely left to find their own ways of coping. Some of this is unavoidable or even necessary, of course, since individual emotional and spiritual needs vary so widely. But even recognition that these issues exist would help, as would some linkage between the physical treatment a woman receives and the emotional/spiritual healing she also pursues.

I was unprepared for the emotional and spiritual impact of my advocacy work. I found that the work I did to create access to information and improved treatment, and the support I could offer women dealing with mental illness related to childbearing, was profoundly healing for me. It fulfilled a need so deep that I knew I could never completely heal until I met it. At the same time, I was dealing with stress and anxiety again, though it was now related to the women I was supporting. I had not learned how to advocate for others while preserving my own strength, or how to balance this new role with my role as a mother.

It took me more than five years, from the time my illness began, to really begin to understand and master this balance. And most of what I learned came not from health care providers, but from my own experience, and from the experiences of others I met along the way who struggled with the same balance. I learned that there is no straight road to recovery. We stumble and fall many times along the way. But we can learn from our experiences each time, and we can find the strength to get up and continue to move forward. From other women working to increase the awareness, treatment, and prevention of mental health issues related to childbearing, I began to learn how to balance giving support to others while nurturing myself. And along the way, I had the support and prayers of my family, friends, and fellow church members. This was a big part of the miracle that is my recovery.

One of the hardest stumbles I encountered came in early 2001, more than ten months after we moved into our new home. My son was 5 years old and attending kindergarten. I was enjoying my expanded role at PSI and felt I was making a real contribution to the organization's work. My husband was doing well at work, and was busy with some additional training required for his job. For this reason, he was away on a two-week business trip. It was the longest period of time he had been away since our son was born.

Neither of us expected any problems when he left. I had been happy and stable for a long time now, and we didn't yet understand just how precarious the balance I was searching for could be.

Then a spider bit my son while he was helping me with some yard work. This was the first insect bite he had received, so I didn't know what to expect. Depending on the species, spider bites can be serious for anyone, and some people are far more sensitive to them than others. I kept a close watch on him, and when he complained, "Mommy, I am hot and sweaty," despite the fact that it was cool outside, I decided it was time for a trip to the emergency room. Fortunately, his reaction was not severe and he recovered quickly.

Any mother would have been concerned when something like this happened to her child, and, of course, the fact that my husband was away intensified the stress. However, in all my natural concern for him, I was not paying attention to myself. Anxiety over his illnesses or injuries had always been a factor in my own illness, something capable of causing, or at least increasing, the chances of a relapse. Part of the balance I would need to learn is how to take care of myself as well as my child when an episode like this occurred.

Shortly afterwards, I received a phone call from a mother who was experiencing serious anxiety and fear surrounding the birth of her child. She needed my support, but I was totally unprepared for the strong impact my concern for her would have on my own emotions. She touched a deep, deep chord in me and it awoke all the old, terrible memories of fear and isolation. It was as if the floor had opened up under me and I was dropped back into all the pain and anguish I had experienced. The reaction I had was so strong that I called my doctor and Jane Honikman for support. I needed help to stabilize my own emotions, and I needed to learn how to detach emotionally from the pain of those I helped—much like doctors become used to doing.

To make matters worse, my normally regular period was now several days late. Since it was already late by the time my stress increased, that seemed unrelated. I began to seriously consider the possibility I was pregnant again. It wouldn't be unwelcome news; Michael and I had begun opening ourselves to the possibility of having another child. But I was also greatly afraid I would suffer a relapse. We were aware that this was a possibility, but we had no real plan for managing the risk; it was not something any of my doctors had discussed with me. The possibility of relapsing now, while my husband was away, terrified me.

Finally, just to make everything perfect, came the night when I realized my son and I might have been exposed to carbon monoxide in our house. I didn't know how much exposure we might have had, or what the threshold for danger was. I started asking questions and researching information. Our family doctor shared my concerns and had me come in for a blood test to check the level of carbon monoxide. Fortunately, the exposure had been minimal, and my son and I were both fine, but the scare had added to my already high stress levels.

Some of the new friends I had made through my work at PSI were military wives. They were used to their husbands being away for protracted periods of time, but I remember them talking about how frequently things seemed to start going wrong as soon as their husbands left. They seemed to regard it as one more fact of life, but this was my first exposure to the phenomenon. I admired their ability to cope, but knew I was now in trouble. For the last several days, I had been unable to eat very much and now I was having trouble sleeping. I called my psychiatric doctor, and she prescribed sleeping pills and put me on bed rest.

With my husband away and an active 5-year-old in the house, this was no easy regime to follow. Earlier in my illness, I probably would have tried to stick it out until Michael got back. Now I made my wellbeing a priority and asked for help. I had accepted the fact that unless I took care of myself, I could not take care of my son, and I could not support the women I so much wanted to help. It was a major step for me and fortunately I now had good friends who understood the need and were more than willing to help. They brought meals to us and helped entertain my son while I rested.

It was during this period I learned just how deeply my illness had impacted my son when he was a baby and a toddler. Even during the worst periods of my illness, Michael and I had made the care and wellbeing of our son our highest priority. We did everything we could to ensure that our son always felt safe and loved, but there was no way we could shield him from being separated from his mother for long periods of time. We had to hope that he was too young for this to have done much damage. Unfortunately, there was a limit to how much we could protect him.

One night, when things had settled down a bit and I was beginning to feel better, I sat down to spend some time with my son. As he cuddled with me on my lap, I reassured him that I was there for him, and that I wasn't going to go away. I told him that things were going to be okay.

I got a reaction I hadn't expected. He became sad, so sad that he took one of the couch pillows and held it in front of his face.

"Why are you doing that?" I asked him softly. "What's the matter?"

"I don't want you to see me crying," he sniffed through his tears.

I kissed him. "Why not?" I asked. "Why are you crying?"

"I remember crying and wanting you, not Daddy," he said.

All I could do was hold him closely, and let him know how much I loved him. I couldn't give him back all the time together we had lost. As a mother, this breaks my heart; as an advocate, it makes me more determined. Every day I see, a little more clearly, how great an impact mental illness related to childbearing has on women and their families.

Despite the difficulties I had encountered, I was proud of how well I had managed. I had been proactive and made the decisions I had to make to avoid a major episode. I was horrified that I had stumbled again, more than five years after my illness began, but I felt like I'd achieved a victory against odds I'd once imagined were overwhelming.

I was delighted when my husband returned from his trip. I had missed him terribly, and our house felt much more peaceful and homelike with his return. I told him what had happened, of course. Beside the fact that he needed to know what had gone on, I wanted to share my victory with him. Well, he was much more concerned about my condition than impressed with my victory. Considering what he had been through in the past, I could hardly blame him, but I did think he was missing an important milestone. I hoped that with the passage of a little time, he would understand what I had achieved.

Soon after his return, he accompanied me to see my doctor. During the visit, I noticed a shift in emphasis. We were back to the, "What is wrong with Jennifer?" model of care. My doctor spoke primarily to my husband rather than to me, as if I were a child or a pet, rather than a responsible participant in my own care. I noticed this with other doctors as well, but I wasn't really aware how pervasive the problem had become until I began to gather my medical records in preparation for writing this book. One event, relatively minor in scope, seemed to me to set me back to the beginning in the eyes of the doctor now responsible for my treatment. As a result of this, what seemed like a victory to me caused Michael to begin questioning my recovery.

There is a great confusion and a general lack of knowledge about psychosis, in particular, and mental health, in general—even among health care professionals. Sometimes I wonder if the only people who actually do understand psychosis are those who have gone through it. Psychosis doesn't make you stupid or unable to take responsibility for yourself. It does often make you delusional, but once these symptoms are managed, people who suffer from psychosis are usually as capable of self-care as people who suffer from appendicitis. In fact, the more they are encouraged to take on the responsibility of self-care, and the more knowledge they have about how to do this, the better the results are likely to be.

By June 2001, I was doing well. I had a part-time flexible job working as an assistant to a pharmaceutical recruiter. I continued my work as a volunteer coordinator with PSI. One week before I was to leave for California to attend my first annual PSI conference, Andrea Yates drowned her five children in Houston, Texas. She suffered from both postpartum depression and postpartum psychosis. It was an enormous national tragedy, and suddenly, everybody was talking about postpartum mental illness. The media frenzy was unbelievable. The coverage was sensational, and much of what was presented about mental illness related to childbearing was either dangerously incomplete or simply incorrect. It was a disturbing picture of just how ignorant our society actually was when it came to mental illness.

Along with the rest of the country, I was horrified by the tragic event, but I think a good part of my shock came from things that would not have occurred to people unfamiliar with mental illness surrounding childbearing. As more details about Andrea's life began to emerge, I was appalled to realize how extensive her history of illness was, and how inadequate her treatment had been. She'd been through several pregnancies with a previous history of postpartum depression. No one apparently had either warned her of the risks during a subsequent pregnancy, or worked with her to manage that risk during her subsequent pregnancies. Things did not appear to have improved much since I became ill in 1996. It grieved me to realize how preventable this tragedy was.

Though I had no way to prove it, of course, I also suspected her spiritual beliefs and welfare had not been considered during treatment. After the fact, the media made them part of the story—or at least part of the cautionary tale they created to demonize Andrea and her husband.

Predictably, opinions about what should happen to Andrea varied greatly depending on whether or not the person holding the opinion knew anything at all about mental illness surrounding childbearing. People who did know something about it were generally grieved for the family and had compassion for Andrea. Those who didn't know anything wanted the harshest penalties as quickly as possible. During the PSI conference, I would learn that the organization's board members, who had spoken out publicly on Andrea's behalf, were receiving death threats. At that time, PSI had already existed for 14 years and had worked tirelessly to increase public awareness of mental illness related to childbearing, and the fact that women who suffer from them typically do not receive adequate care. During those dark days in June, it seemed the country had actually made little progress in understanding or treating mental illness related to childbearing. Now the country was paying attention, but it was the media's sensationalized, often inaccurate, coverage that was shaping the public perception of these illnesses.

Although I did not recognize it at the time, I think, looking back, that my husband found the controversy surrounding the Andrea Yates case more stressful than I did. We had started a new life when we moved, and only close family and friends knew our history with postpartum psychosis. After the tragedy, my husband had to listen to people at work voice their opinions of what should happen to Andrea for drowning her children. None of them could understand why her husband could stand by her after the tragedy. Having no direct experience, they could not understand how her illness could have precipitated her action, or that she could have sincerely believed she was saving her children. In fact, some of them apparently regarded postpartum psychosis as a trendy legal excuse. Experience, of course, had given Michael a far greater understanding of illnesses like postpartum psychosis; he could easily imagine just how ill she'd been that day and the kind of disordered thinking that had driven her actions. Explaining that to the people around him, though, was another matter entirely. The tragedy brought back some very painful memories that had just begun to fade. He wasn't willing to go into them simply to educate the curious. I could hardly blame him.

The PSI conference in California became a pivotal event for me. It was my first opportunity to meet with other advocates from around the country, and I learned a great deal about what other people and organizations were doing. Even without the dramatic lessons the Andrea Yates tragedy provided, I began to realize just how little progress the United States had made in preventing and treating mental illnesses related to childbearing, and raising public awareness of them. We had so much work left to do, and it looked like it was going to be an uphill climb.

At the time, I remember asking myself, "Why aren't our leaders supporting laws to address the need for education, further research, and funding?" I couldn't imagine how anybody could oppose an effort to prevent needless suffering. At the time, I was just beginning my advocacy. I now know a great deal more about entrenched bureaucracies, the inertia of the status quo, and a political system driven by deep-pocketed special interest groups. But I still think it's a good question. Why aren't they routinely working to address all needless suffering, not just the needless suffering of women experiencing mental illness related to childbearing? Why aren't we all doing that as a country?

Later that year, another tragedy would sear itself onto all of our minds and begin some new discussions about how we treat each other in the community. On September 11, 2001 terrorists hijacked four commercial aircraft. They flew two of the planes into the World Trade Center. One they flew into the Pentagon. The fourth crashed in Pennsylvania after brave passengers attempted to take back control of the plane from the hijackers. Almost 3,000 people died that day, and as a country we are still dealing with our grief over the losses, care for first-responders and others who have developed illnesses related to the event, and the consequences of our national response to the tragedy.

In addition to the more obvious lessons from this terrible event, I've gained a few specific insights that come from my own experience, and what I see as parallels between the Andrea Yates tragedy and the events of September 11th.

As I write this, more than 12 years have passed. Once again we've lost sight of the motto that bound us together through that dreadful time, "United We Stand." We have gone back to divisive politics with a vengeance and lost sight of the welfare of the country as a whole. We don't take care of one another. As many people now recognize, there were things we could have done to prevent the tragedy on September 11th. If you consult various people, you'll get various lists of just exactly what those things are, but there is a consensus that what we failed to do had grave consequences for our nation.

The tragedy that happened in June of that year was also preventable. We know what happened to Andrea Yates and her family because that event was unusually horrific and highly covered. We don't see the suffering that other women experience with mental illnesses related to childbearing. The tragedies that result from these illnesses don't make headlines, but are just as preventable.

God has blessed me with a strong man for a husband, one who has helped me through life's stormiest currents. He stood by me while I was sick when most men would not have. Now he wanted to put all the dark days behind us. He wanted us to live the kind of life we'd both envisioned when we first married. I wanted to help prevent a tragedy like Andrea Yates from ever happening again. That tragedy had changed my life forever and from it I gained a new commitment as an advocate. I was determined to do my part to take care of others in my community, in this very specific way. As I became more involved in my work as an activist though, I failed to realize just how much Michael wanted to put my illness behind us. This would create some new challenges for us, as well as present us with opportunities to grow in our relationship.

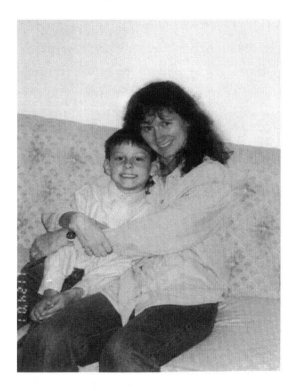

My son and I on his 6th birthday in 2001 with our strong bond rebuilt despite our lost time together.

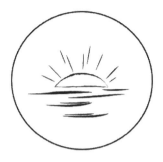

Chapter 13

A New Journey Begins

Since the birth of my son, sleep had been a major challenge for me. I could generally fall asleep, but sleeping deeply for the length of time it takes for the body to repair itself often eluded me. Some of my sleeplessness was undoubtedly caused by the stress of new motherhood and the needs of an infant in the house, but some was clearly related to the onset of my illness. When I am sleep deprived, there is a good chance that I will become fearful and maybe that I will start hearing and seeing things.

Since the onset of my illness, my doctors had managed my sleep problems by prescribing sleeping pills. as needed, along with other drugs, such as anti-psychotic medication. After my first psychotic episode, I was prescribed a powerful anti-psychotic drug that had been on the market for a long time. It was effective at preventing any recurrence of symptoms. The problem was that the side effects were terrible. I was glad when, prior to our move in 1999, my doctor had allowed me to go off of it. That left me with only one drug that I took regularly.

All this changed after the problems that began in 2001. For one thing, I had become much more proactive in my own care. For another, that episode had persuaded me that I needed to make some changes. Finally, I was frustrated by the fact that medication was the only tool I was offered to help regulate my sleeplessness and stress, and prevent a relapse of my illness. I told my doctor that I wanted to change my medications and asked her to explore the options with me.

As a result of the symptoms I was having, our discussion led to her recommending that we re-introduce an anti-psychotic. This made me extremely apprehensive; the side effects of the last anti-psychotic I'd been on had been devastating. I told her that I never wanted to go back on that drug again, and she said, "I would never give that to my patients." She explained that there were newer drugs available that were just as effective and had far fewer side effects. I'd been seeing her for about six months at that point and trusted her enough that I overcame my reluctance and agreed to this course of treatment. What I've learned since then, and still find troubling, is that patients are still prescribed older medications, knowing the severity of their side effects, despite the availability of new alternatives that are far easier to tolerate.

She had also prescribed a drug that would replace my regular medication. She explained that it would have fewer side effects and do a better job managing the symptoms triggered by the additional stress. Almost immediately after I began the new medication, I had an adverse reaction to the pills, so she switched the prescription from a capsule to a time-release tablet. That seemed to work well except that the only tablets available were 600 mg which were too sedating for me. After more discussion, and with my doctor's agreement, I began taking the pills every other day. That worked well and my energy levels were restored.

I was pleased to have a doctor who respected me and who would allow me to be a partner in my own treatment. In my experience, this is rare good fortune. However, I still felt there was something missing. I had been taking prescribed medications since the onset of my illness in 1996. They were intended to treat my symptoms, or prevent them from reoccurring. But as far as I could tell, they didn't actually address the underlying cause. The part of the puzzle I was missing then, and didn't learn until much later, was that my regular drug was actually a mood-stabilizer. These are prescribed long-term for people who suffer the kind of chemical imbalances that cause such things as bipolar disorder. But none of my doctors had ever discussed this with me. I'd had no history of mental illness before my son's birth, so I still believed there was no reason not to expect to regain my previous good health. The idea that I would be taking long-term medication simply to control my symptoms, instead of a program to address the underlying causes of my symptoms, did not sit well with me. It seemed like a good idea for the pharmaceutical industry, but a poor one for a patient.

So I began to look around for alternatives to the standard model of treatment. I made my first forays into alternative medicine in 2002. At that time, I began to have very heavy, painful menstrual periods. The only other time I had experienced this problem was before I became pregnant with my son, but after his birth my periods returned to normal. I began to explore some natural methods that would more gently help my body return to its natural rhythm. I was pleased with the results, and the experience gave me a much more favorable opinion of alternative medicine than I previously had.

When my sister Marie's fiancé was diagnosed with cancer at about the same time, his diagnosis motivated me to explore alternative medicine in depth. I was impressed with its holistic philosophy—to support the health of the entire person: physically, emotionally, mentally, and spiritually as a patient healed from an illness or trauma. It was a concise statement of what I felt had been missing from my own treatment from the beginning.

Unfortunately, what I learned came too late to help Marie's fiancé, and I set aside looking into holistic medicine as we dealt with the grief of his passing. After several months, I was compelled to learn even more about it. Even though I was now on medication with far fewer side effects, I was dissatisfied with my prospects. I continued to believe that I did not need medication for the rest of my life simply designed to fight off my symptoms. I yearned to heal completely and wanted to undertake a comprehensive health regime that would preserve my health and prevent the occurrence of illness in the future. At this point, I didn't see that Western medicine offered me a way to get there.

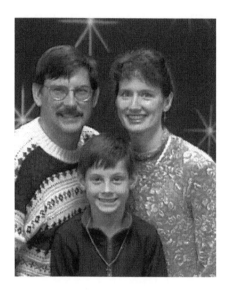

Our family Christmas photo in 2002.

As I learned more about alternative/natural medicine, it became obvious to me that stress is one of the leading causes of illness. I knew, of course, that it had been a major trigger for my own illness. I now began to understand its physical effects on the body, and how these effects undermine the proper balance of body, mind, emotions, and spirit that is necessary for good health. I decided that my first step should be to find a way to better manage my own stress levels. As part of this effort, I was introduced to the practice of Reiki by a woman that was both a nurse and Reiki instructor. I eagerly began to explore this Japanese form of energy healing. Reiki literally means "universal life energy." This is the energy with which martial artists and yoga students (to name a few people) are familiar. It's called *Ki* in Japanese, *Chi* in Chinese, and *Prana* in Hindi. Some Christians refer to it as the energy of the Holy Spirit. It is a very gentle, noninvasive practice that seeks to restore the flow of energy throughout the body. Once blockages to the flow of energy are removed, the body can release stored toxins and the renewed flow of energy revitalizes internal systems. This allows the body's own healing processes to work more efficiently, and relaxes the mind and spirit. I heard testimonies of how effective it was so I started taking a few Reiki sessions myself, which led me to enroll in a Reiki training course.

It was fascinating. I felt as if I had become a student at the Japanese School of Stress Management and Reduction. As the two-month training progressed, I began to feel a peace I had never experienced before. I mastered the symbols and movements and learned to channel the energy through my own body. From the Reiki sessions, I received the practice I could now do on my own. I believed that since I was now able to manage my symptoms, I was completely healed. Through the use of Reiki, I would be able to maintain the balance I needed to stay in good health.

My illness, and especially my near-death experience, had changed my worldview and my spiritual understanding in ways that were difficult to explain to anyone else. Unfortunately, this included my husband, Michael. The doctors had told him that "religiosity"—seen as religious devotion to the extreme—was a symptom of psychosis, so his concern was understandable in regards to my interest in "spiritual pursuits." To him, it would indicate a recurrence of my illness. It is true, of course, that women who suffer from postpartum psychosis often suffer from religious visions, but I viewed mine as something other than simply a symptom. Whatever else the spiritual symptoms of my illness may have been, to me they were an expression of a deep spiritual imbalance I was working to address. My "spiritual pursuits" helped address this imbalance, and one of the ways I did this was through alternative medical practices like Reiki. Michael, whose view had been formed by traditional Western medicine, seemed unconvinced by my belief that this was the best path for me; his perspective, in fact, was that it might prove dangerous. His perspective was formed by a more traditional approach of focusing primarily on medication management. As a result of this difference in opinion, I slowly learned not to discuss my alternative medical practices with my husband. This, I would learn, is not healthy for a marriage.

About a month after I completed my Reiki training, I accepted my first job as a certified postpartum *doula*. According to the DONA International, the word doula comes from an ancient Greek word meaning "a woman who serves." The word is now used to refer to a trained and experienced professional who provides physical, emotional, and informational support to a mother before, during, and soon after birth. She may also provide emotional and practical support throughout the entire postpartum period as well. I was proud to be doing this work and delighted that I had been hired by a wonderful professional couple who were having their first child.

On the morning of what would be my second day of work for the couple, I received a totally unexpected phone call. The house phone rang while I was in my office, but since it didn't ring for long, I figured my husband had answered it. Shortly afterward, Michael called on the intercom and asked me to pick up the phone. When I did, I recognized the voice immediately. It was my sister Elizabeth.

"Mom is gone," she said.

"What?" I screamed. That made no sense at all to me. I knew that Mom was traveling with my brother, David, for Elizabeth's daughter's high school graduation. In fact, I had just talked to Mom the day before, the morning before they began the drive to Maryland. Mom was excited and busy preparing for the trip, so we only spoke briefly. This was unusual for us; I loved talking to my mother and our calls were usually lengthy.

"There was an accident," Elizabeth went on to say. Her words took my breath away and I could feel the ache in my heart. She went on to tell me that less than to two miles from her house, David lost control of the car and Mom was injured. Although her injuries seemed slight initially, her pancreas had actually been severed and she died in surgery. Elizabeth's words now made an awful kind of sense; she really was gone.

At first, I was just angry. This anger turned towards God and the universe in general. My mother had been in excellent health all her life, so I was completely unprepared for this sudden, dramatic loss. But I knew my mother's spiritual beliefs and she raised me to have faith. Though I grieved deeply, and I missed her more with each passing day, I found some comfort in the knowledge that she was at peace in heaven. The night after her funeral, I experienced the first restful night's sleep I'd had since I learned of her death. The next day, I shared this with my sisters, Anne and Lynette. They'd had the same experience, and that night both of them were finally able to sleep peacefully as well. Mom had given us a final gift. It didn't lessen our grief, but believing she was at peace helped us bear our loss.

My husband returned home after my mother's funeral, but my son and I stayed in Pennsylvania with my family. I already had plans to attend the PSI annual conference in New York City. It was scheduled to begin about a month after Mom's death, and she had planned to attend. She had been very supportive and proud of my volunteer work, so I knew that she would still want me to go.

Shortly before the conference, though, my spiritual life took a turn for the worse. Although I was still using Reiki for stress and relaxation, my experience was changing. Now I began to sense spiritual presences around me as I channeled the energy through my body. This was a new dimension to my practice, and I didn't really understand what I was experiencing. I longed for my mother even more. She had been my spiritual "guru," and she'd always been just a phone call away when I sought her guidance and opinions. None of the presences or energies I had encountered seemed to threaten me, but I missed being able to talk to her about what I was experiencing. I continued to pray and, though grieved, my spirit was able to remain peaceful.

My arrival in New York City was exciting. This was my first trip to the city, so in addition to spending time with my fellow PSI volunteers, I planned to spend some time exploring the city. The first few days went according to plan and I had a good time, but I also noticed that my period was a few days late. I had to consider the possibility that I was pregnant, so I called my doctor to ask if the medication I was taking was safe during pregnancy. It was not a surprise when he told me that it was not advisable to take it during the first six weeks. I was torn; I was already beginning to feel a surge in my hormones. I was sure something was happening; I just wasn't completely sure what it was.

At that point I truly believed I was miscarrying, though I'll never know for sure since it was so early. Whatever was going on, it concerned me enough to share with those that knew me at the conference. Before the conference ended, one of the attendees, a leading perinatal mental health expert, arranged for me to be seen at New York Presbyterian Hospital. Everything was handled very discreetly and professionally; I took a taxi to the hospital where I was seen by two doctors, including an expert in the field of mental health related to childbearing.

It was a lengthy emergency room visit and during his consultation he told me that I was most likely suffering from bipolar disorder, postpartum onset. Finally, more than six years after the onset of postpartum psychosis, I had an expert diagnosis of the condition that seemed to be causing my recurring symptoms. He said there was medication available that I could take to help balance my chemistry. He also explained that thyroid disorders can sometimes cause symptoms that are easily mistaken for postpartum mental illness and advised me to see an endocrinologist to rule out any other underlying or contributing medical issues. Unfortunately, even today, many doctors don't routinely order thyroid screenings for postpartum women, and that omission can cause a world of needless pain.

The incident caught me and everyone else around me by surprise. I had believed I had entirely recovered from my illness, but what happened in New York City showed me that this might not actually be true. Having a consultation by a specialist in the field of mental health related to childbearing revealed to me that traditional medicine may have to play a role in my healing. His diagnosis was a big piece of the puzzle that had been missing. I began to accept that, from now on, I would most likely have to combine traditional and alternative medical strategies to maintain the physical, mental, emotional, and spiritual balance I had been seeking.

Michael had already arrived at his parents' home in Pennsylvania, as was the plan, so that the two of us, along with our son, could travel home after I returned from the conference. The problem now was that I was in an emergency room in New York City. So Michael and my brother, David, decided to drive together on the two-hour trip to pick me up from the hospital. It was a comfort to me to see them when they arrived. Arriving back in Pennsylvania brought me peace. As a family we'd suffered a tremendous loss just a month ago, and now, with what had just happened to me, I began to see that the stresses in my marriage to Michael were beginning to accumulate. The mental illness, along with the many hospitalizations and physical setbacks, had caused a strain on our marital relationship. Michael had remained strong, and his love for me and our son never wavered. But trying to understand what was going on with me, while holding down a job and helping to care for me and our son, was causing a rift; we couldn't go back to how it was before the onset of postpartum psychosis, so we were having to adjust to what it had now become. It would take some time to heal the rift that had arisen between us.

Once I got back to Florida, I followed up with an endocrinologist as the doctor from New York Presbyterian Hospital had suggested. I saw the endocrinologist several times and he ordered a series of tests. The tests revealed that my blood sugar levels fluctuated more than normal, and the doctor suggested that I monitor them. My cortisol levels were also a little high, but not high enough to cause concern. Eventually, he would rule out any underlying physical causes for my condition. So I had an official diagnosis: bipolar disorder, postpartum onset. Well, I had wanted a diagnosis, but I wasn't expecting this. I thought that knowing exactly what was wrong could help me heal. And it did, eventually, but first I had to come to terms with a harsh reality. Bipolar disorder doesn't go away and leaves you with a permanent label. My journal entry from July 24, 2003 sums up where I stood.

> ….not only did the doctor's diagnosis leave me with the inability to ever get affordable insurance coverage on my own, it has left its mark on my marriage. A mark I doubt can be repaired…I have discovered that bipolar is a classification of mood disorders and that the real cause is not known. It may be convenient for the medical community to make such a diagnosis, but oh how detrimental it can be to receive it.

By August 2003, I recognized that there were untreated wounds in our marriage. In September, my husband brought up divorce for the first time. He seemed to dismiss the idea when I reminded him, in front of our son, that our wedding vows said, "for better or worse," but I knew my prayers for our marriage would need to continue. I asked God to heal our marriage. I asked Him for strength, patience, and passion to do all that I believed He wanted me to do. I asked Him to shed His love and healing light on our family.

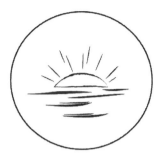

Chapter 14

More to the Story

In November 2003, my husband was scheduled to leave for a month-long, work-related trip to another country. In the past, the longest trip he had ever been assigned was two weeks long. The trip came at an inopportune time as well. With the help of counseling, Michael and I had done a lot of work on our marriage and things were improving for us. It didn't seem like a good time to interrupt that progress. There was no other choice though; it was a necessary trip for his job. Since things were going well overall, I did not expect any problems while he was gone. After all, I had a good support system in place and I was healthy and stable. I continued to monitor my blood sugar levels as recommended by the endocrinologist. He had also referred me to a dietician who taught me how to use nutrition to regulate my sugars, without additional medication. Still things happen in their own timing, whether or not you are prepared for them. I took Michael to the airport, asking God to keep him safe as well as to continue to give me peace, comfort, and strength while he was away.

Things went well for the initial month my husband was away. It was after his trip got extended for two weeks that things started to unravel causing sparks that would ultimately cause everything to go up in flames. Just ten days before Michael's scheduled return, the first spark contributing to the fire ignited. A local controversy began when the school board in our community decided to rezone. As often seems to happen with these kinds of things, the zoning was handled pretty haphazardly and without much regard to the existing school population. My son, along with many other children in our community, would be forced to go to a school outside the community.

Naturally, parents were concerned. We liked the current school our children attended, so parents were upset by the fact that the board did not consult with those who would be affected by the situation prior to the decision to make the change. Parents were notified of the rezoning when letters were sent home from school with the children. I, along with other parents, began to organize a protest to the change, and since I already had some experience as a community activist, I quickly found myself assuming a prominent role. I was happy to do it, of course; I felt this was a critical issue to my son's future—as did the other parents. However, the increased stress began to impact my sleep patterns.

In addition to all of this, I continued my work as a volunteer coordinator for PSI and had recently been commissioned as a Stephen Minister. A Stephen Minister is a layperson who provides emotional and spiritual support for other members of the congregation. Much of this support comes from employing one of the strongest support tools available: listening without interruption. That type of support is something that people may rarely receive and it can be profoundly healing. When combined with encouragement and empathy, the results are powerful. However, the role of a Stephen Minister is a serious, long-term commitment. The training provided me with the knowledge that listening is an art requiring skill and compassion. Although I loved both of my roles as a coordinator and a minister, I began to feel a pull on my strength that silently ignited the second spark of the ensuing fire.

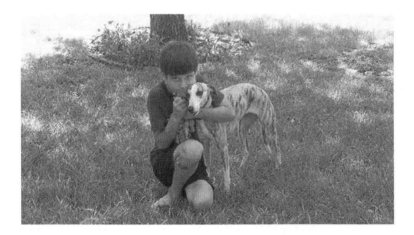

My son and his dog in 2003, the same year my mom died and the idea to write this book was birthed.

The "small flames began to flicker," as I gave emotional support to a neighbor, whom I had grown close to since moving to the community three years ago. Recently, she and her husband separated. They were trying to reconcile, but in the midst of all of this, he had to deploy for several months. The status of their marriage and future relationship was completely unknown, causing her to have much doubt when he left. Her stress level was high with his departure and the uncertainty of his commitment to both her and to their children.

On the same night her husband left for deployment, I was on the phone with her when our phone call was interrupted by another call. She put me on hold for a few moments while she took the call, and then returned to tell me that the call had come from a man at our church who had begun to pursue her romantically. She did not encourage or welcome his attention. In fact, she made this clear to him. She felt uncomfortable with the situation, and the more she described it, I was as well.

Rather than confront the man, I consulted with another one of my close friends. I valued this friend's opinion, so I sought her advice. After we finished our discussion and prayed for direction in the situation, it became clear to me what to do. Since this man was an active member of the church my neighbor and I both attended, I should bring what was happening to the attention of the senior pastor. My neighbor did not feel comfortable enough to discuss it with him directly, so I would speak to him on her behalf.

Since my son had a scheduled music lesson at the church in a few days, I decided I would wait to talk to the senior pastor, in person, during my son's lesson. Unfortunately, on that day the senior pastor was not there. I did get to speak with him briefly via telephone. He told me that he was unavailable for the rest of the day, but if I felt comfortable doing so, I could talk to the associate pastor. This wasn't ideal, as I did not know him as well, but I thought it best to address the situation as soon as possible. I proceeded to explain to the associate pastor my neighbor's situation. I also shared with him that the man who was pursuing her was from our church. Although the man was someone she was familiar with and seemed harmless, I went on to tell him that this man was currently going through a divorce so it was likely that he was in need of spiritual counseling and emotional support himself. At the close of our conversation, I said, "I believe that there is a spirit of divorce affecting the church." I went on to explain that I thought the spirit was preventing the church from sanctifying and strengthening marriages among its congregation. Our conversation ended with little input from him. Actually, he seemed to not understand what I was telling him. As I left his office, I asked him to please pass this information on to the senior pastor so the matter would be addressed.

Two days later, I went to an event at the church, so I took the opportunity to speak to the senior pastor myself with hopes of learning how the matter was being addressed. Since I was not sure how much information was relayed to him by the associate pastor, I reiterated the situation to him.

I was soon dismayed when he seemed as unconcerned as the associate pastor had been. In fact, he simply asked, "Are you taking your medication?" His question frustrated me, since it was none of his business. At the time, I simply wrote it off as a heavy-handed form of concern. So I did answer the question, telling him, yes, I was taking my medication. My church community was aware of my history with postpartum psychosis as I had shared my testimony in front of the church back in 2002. This pastor was not in leadership at the church in 2002. Even though he knew me personally and I was active in the church, I did not feel it appropriate for him to even bring the question up to me. Even though I did answer his question, I did not mention to him that I was currently between doctors. Our health insurance company had recently changed and my doctor was not a provider for the new insurance plan. I still needed to find a doctor who was a provider with the new insurance. Our finances were tight, and I could not afford to continue to see my doctor because I would have to pay the full office visit charge, not just the office visit copay amount. Since I was still in professional counseling and had a supply of my regular medication, I did not think finding a new doctor was urgent. I wanted to take my time and find someone I could connect with as well as I had connected with my previous doctor. And anyway, the whole issue was irrelevant to our conversation.

Before our conversation ended, I did mention that it had been a couple of days since I had heard from my husband, who was still out of the country. Michael and I had been able to speak regularly up until this point. I did express that

I had some concern that I had not heard from him, which was causing additional stress. With Michael expected home by the end of the week, and the fact that the past ten days had been particularly stressful, I asked the senior pastor if the church might be able to provide me with some practical support. I was desperately in need of some help in catching up with many of the household chores.

After I returned home from the meeting, I decided to check in on my neighbor and see how she was doing. I tried to call her and couldn't get through, so I went over to her house. She told me that she was fine, but that she was having trouble with her phone. Oddly, it seemed every number she dialed connected to the wrong number. I tried placing a call myself, and the same thing happened to me. We were unable to think of any possible reason for this to happen, so it left us both feeling uneasy. In addition, she started discovering a few unusual things since her husband left on deployment. I did not know exactly what she had discovered, but she was clearly disturbed by what she'd found and worried about her husband's state of mind.

The more we talked the more uneasy we both became, and I remembered that our house alarm system had begun having some problems. Suddenly, I didn't want to go back home alone. I called another neighbor, who is a professional builder, and asked him to meet me at my house. I explained some of the situation to him and told him that, under the circumstances, we felt a little vulnerable as single moms. He offered to come back the next day and check out the alarm system. I agreed with relief and thanked him for his help.

I simply did not feel safe being home alone—not at all because I was suicidal, or homicidal, or hearing voices, or anything else of that nature. Earlier in the evening when my neighbor and I began to wonder if her husband had orchestrated some of the odd things that were going on, the idea that he may have done so made me concerned for our safety.

The thought crossed my mind that my neighbor's husband may have been behind the strange things that were occurring at her house. Even if it seemed unlikely, my state of mind at that point became subject to consider that there were individuals who may have evil intent toward my neighbor, as well as myself. Whether rational or not, my belief was genuine.

My feeling of uneasiness about being alone in the house did not subside. Since I did not know when my church would respond to my request for practical support, I thought to contact a woman I knew from the community prayer and praise group I attended. She was single and seemed to be a caring, dependable person. I thought she might have the time to provide me with some practical assistance. I was able to reach her immediately. She said she was available to help and could spend the night as well. Knowing that there would be another adult in the house made me feel safe immediately.

She arrived at 8:30 p.m., just after I tucked my son into bed. My son had been upset that he was once again not able to talk to his dad before he went to bed. He was missing him terribly. In fact, earlier that day my son actually asked if he could stay home from school for the day. My son loved school, so that was a very unusual request. As I reflected on our last telephone conversation on Friday, I remembered how Michael had told me he'd run into a communist in the former Soviet country he was visiting for his job training. That gave me some concern at the time, but Michael assured me there was absolutely nothing to worry about. I agreed that he was probably right—former communists must be pretty thick on the ground there—but now it was Monday night and still no word from him. Now I had concern. I told myself I was grasping at straws; the simpler truth is that I had been under unusual stress for the past week and just wanted to hear his voice.

I decided to call the retired Air Force friend that Michael told me to contact if there were any problems. As the wife of a corporate contract employer for the Air Force, this was the only avenue before me if I needed to contact him. When I spoke to Michael's friend, he assured me things were probably fine. Maybe he was aware that Michael was at a training location that prevented him from communicating with me for several days, an important piece of information that I would not learn for another week or two. It was 8:30 p.m. when the woman from church had arrived at the house. I felt so relaxed that at 10:00 p.m., I took my medication as usual and went to bed. At 2:30 a.m., I woke from a sound sleep feeling as if I was suffocating. Then I heard the back door open and got up to investigate. It turned out to be the lady from the church group letting out our dog. Through the back door, I watched as the dog raced down the stairs of the deck into the yard. She went straight to the bird aviary and began barking ferociously. Since our dog rarely barks, I thought this highly unusual. I went out to investigate. I couldn't see what, if anything, she was barking at, but I calmed her down and coaxed her back into the house. I figured that a snake got into the aviary to threaten the birds.

Needless to say, I was wide awake by this point and now, as I looked at the church group lady, I began to see how oddly she was dressed. She was wearing a black sweat suit and ski cap even though it was not cold outside. In addition, she'd brought a few things into the house that I found unusual, including an alarm clock that ticked very loudly and a binder that she had showed me earlier that included some information she'd collected about me. Suddenly, it began to dawn on me how little I knew about this woman. Originally, I was comfortable inviting her into my home, but now I realized the only fact I knew about her is that she normally attended the Church of Latter Day Saints. When she began attending our group, she shared that she was unhappy at her church and came upon our church as a result of her search for spiritual support.

Now I felt a sense of panic at her presence in my house. I discreetly called a dear friend. I explained the situation, we prayed together and I shared with her that my fear was so great that I thought I should call the police for assistance. She agreed that this was a good idea and told me that she was going to drive to my house as soon as possible.

I made the call to the police as quietly as I could. Even before they arrived, my friend did. I felt some relief. A moment later, the police arrived. They handled the situation very calmly and professionally. I politely asked the woman to leave my home, while the police officers stood inside the front door of my house. She was compliant and as she left, she quietly acknowledged that she knew she was dressed oddly. The officers stayed a few minutes longer as I further explained the situation. They understood and advised me that, in the future, it would be wise not to invite people I didn't know into my house.

I acknowledged that this was a risk I hadn't really considered, but explained that I was generally a positive, supportive person who looked for the best in people. I told them that since I had been under considerable stress, I had sought support from my church. This woman had been the only person available. Though I did not know her particularly well, she had always struck me as kind. It did not occur to me until that night that she possibly was in need of mental health services herself. I remembered that in the past she had mentioned that she was having financial difficulties and had no access to health care. After she was asked to leave by the police, she drove away and I do not know what happened to her after she left.

By 3:30 or 4:00 a.m., after the officers left, I went back to bed. At 6:00 a.m., my normal time, I got up to begin my day and began processing what had happened over the past few days. In doing so, I realized that on the last few occasions I picked up my son from school, the car line was unusually short. In fact, I recalled several parents pulling their cars out of the line because their children did not emerge from the school building at the appropriate time. This was highly unusual and had never happened in the two and a half years my son had attended the school; usually the pickup of children after classes ended was managed very efficiently. I began to wonder what was going on.

When my 8-year-old son got up at 7:00 a.m., I asked him if anything unusual had been going on at school. My son, who usually had no problem talking to me, suddenly seemed reluctant to say anything. Of course, I reassured him that he could talk to me about anything, and slowly he began to describe some incidents that made me wonder if there might be a real problem at the school. I decided to call my son's pediatrician for advice. Since his previous pediatrician had retired in September, he had a new doctor and we'd seen him only once before. I called the doctor's office and his receptionist advised me to bring my son in to see the doctor so we could discuss the situation with him. She told me that this was the first step in initiating any investigation of the school.

I agreed, made the appointment for 1:15 that afternoon, and then called the school to tell them that my son had a doctor's appointment and would not be attending that day. Actually, I had been trying since 8:00 a.m. to call them, without success. This too was highly unusual. It was almost 9:00 a.m. before someone at the school answered. When I asked if everything was all right, the person on the other end of the phone said that things were fine.

I was concerned enough to tell my neighbor what was going on and she decided to go with us to the doctor. Since her older son also attended the school, I asked the doctor to include her in the consultation. He did not object to this.

My son told the doctor the same things he had told me. What emerged from the conversation was puzzling, but in my mind it revealed that something bad was happening at the school. First, my son told the doctor there were bad guys at the school. He went on to say that the "bad guys at school are big kids." From the sound of it there was some bullying going on, but when gently pressed for details my son said that the principal and the assistant principal would "come down" and take turns yelling, "You're it!" He didn't know the reason behind what they said.

Next, my son told the doctor that the TV in the school had been playing alien movies and that "they"—he and some of the other children, I presume—"had to go in to the bathrooms." I thought that must mean that he had been frightened by the movies, but at this point my neighbor mentioned that her son had talked about "alien movies" as well. My son told the doctor that the children had been asked to draw pictures of the aliens.

Finally, my son said that the children were offered brownies and candy. We limit sweets in our house, but my son confessed that he could not resist the brownies, though he refused everything else. This was the part he was most upset about. I assured him that I was not angry with him and that although we didn't eat many sweets, I knew they could be hard to turn down.

I was disturbed by what I heard. Even with the limited details my son offered, and there didn't seem to be anything overtly threatening going on, it was clear that he had been made very uncomfortable by what he had experienced. The doctor appeared disturbed by what my son said as well, but, as it would turn out, for an entirely different reason.

My son was a happy, intelligent child. He was, and is, strong willed—a trait he gets from both of his parents—but he understood reasoning quite well. And he knew the difference between right and wrong, and between making up stories and telling the truth. However odd the incidents he described sounded, I was sure he was telling the truth. But I'm not sure that the doctor understood that. When he said, at the close of the appointment, that he would contact someone he knew and trusted "at the department," he led me to believe this was the first step to launching an investigation into what was happening at the school. He didn't specify what "department" he meant, and I, trusting him, didn't ask for clarification.

In hindsight, I see that I should have taken my son to a therapist instead of his pediatrician. A trained therapist would have been much better equipped to deal with the situation and would have helped my son express his fears. Unfortunately, the therapist he had seen when he entered kindergarten was no longer in private practice. My son suffered severe separation anxiety that could be traced back to the trauma of my early hospitalizations. However, he responded well to counseling and the therapist had told us that she didn't need to see her unless a new problem emerged. Since that had been three years ago, we'd had no reason to find a new therapist.

The step I took in taking my son to his pediatrician ultimately cost my family dearly. The "flames" that had begun to burn as a result of those earlier "sparks" now became a fiery inferno. It turned out that the "department" he called was the Department of Children and Families (DCF). The doctor told us to stay until "the investigator" arrived so that he could talk to my son. Of course, I agreed to this. I trusted my son's doctor. I thought he believed my son and was continuing the steps necessary to protect my son and discover what was happening at the school. I never imagined what the final outcome would be.

When the investigator arrived, he spoke with both my son and me alone. My son repeated the same information he had told both the doctor and me. My son was not asked any questions unrelated to his experience at school. Naturally, when the investigator asked us to go to the waiting room while he looked into the situation further, we did.

After what seemed like hours, the investigator and the doctor came into the waiting room. The doctor looked uncomfortable and a bit shaken as the investigator proceeded to tell me that my son was going to be removed from my care.

I couldn't believe it. I had done nothing but try to get help for my child, and now I was being treated like a negligent mother. My son immediately began to cry and jumped into my lap for protection. "No, no," he sobbed, over and over. To me, the trauma brought upon my son as a result of what these two men were doing was the worst part of it all.

It was unconscionable, but I was finally beginning to understand what was going on. I had been working with PSI since 2001, and had begun to build a reputation as an advocate since my first national media exposure in February 2002. At the time, the response had been largely positive and I felt like I'd made a contribution to educating people about postpartum psychosis, the relatively rare illness, from which I suffered. However, it's also true that people had learned a part of my story. I'd never considered that there might be a personal risk to me and my family in going public. Now I was beginning to experience, in my own community, the very real consequences of the public's fear and ignorance of mental illness. During the time we'd spent in the waiting room, my pastor had unexpectedly arrived. I'd been astonished to see him, since I had no idea how he knew where I was, but he'd been a welcome presence during the long wait. Now I began to wonder if he had been part of this.

The inspector allowed my pastor to drive all of us back to the house in my van. As we left the office, the investigator said to me, "When you get to your house, there will be officers there waiting to talk to you. Most likely, you will be forced to go to a psychiatric hospital."

By the time we arrived at my house it was dark outside, but as we approached my house, I could see the flashing lights of two police cruisers. What the investigator said was coming true. I felt myself swell with panic. One of the police cars blocked the street and the other one was parked in front of the house. The pastor parked the van in the driveway. I was the last to walk into my house, but as I did, two police officers followed me. One of the officers, wearing a green uniform came with me as I went into my bedroom to listen to the messages on my answering machine. I could not believe that there were twelve messages. Why were there so many? I never had that many messages. As I sat on the bed to listen to the messages, the officer came over to sit beside me. I felt a violating fear. His presence made me so uncomfortable and I did not trust him, so I left the room quickly.

When I went out to the living room, I saw that my neighbor was trying to prepare food for the children. Now a different officer that I hadn't seen until now was there. This officer was wearing a blue uniform rather than a green one as had the other officer I'd left in my bedroom. This officer had stood inside the house, having entered through the garage door and proceeded to walk down the hallway towards the master bedroom. I followed him. He walked right into the bathroom, where he began searching the medicine cabinet. He grabbed a bottle of pills in the cabinet and said, "You are not taking your medication." I told him it was an old prescription bottle. I tried to explain that I no longer took those pills since I was now taking a different medication. My explanation made no difference. He simply refused to listen to me as he stormed out of the house. I did not understand what was happening. I looked around the kitchen and went into the living room, but now only the investigator and two officers, one with a green uniform and the other with a blue one were there. "Where did everyone go?" I asked. The investigator looked up from the chair he sat in holding a folder on his lap and said, "Your son will be in the temporary custody of your neighbor until you have been evaluated."

"Can I at least say goodbye to my son?" I asked. The investigator began to agree, but the officer in the green uniform intervened, refusing to allow it.

"I will go voluntarily, if I have to be evaluated," I said. Despite my request, the green uniformed police officer proceeded to handcuff me. I pleaded that I be taken to the hospital in the area located near my therapist. There was no response. I now had fear for my life, so I began to struggle and resist. This only made him tighten the handcuffs; leaving me with a scar on my wrist to remind me of that dreadful day. He dragged me out of the house and forced me into a squad car. This green uniformed officer began to drive me away.

Before we left, I pleaded that they let me get my cell phone and wallet. My appeal was rejected. Now I was in a panic, gripped with terror. If none of my family or friends knew where I was, anything could happen to me. Even I did not know where I was being taken. I live in a small community, but I knew no one in law enforcement and had no experience with the local hospitals. As it now appeared, my community had turned on me somehow deciding that I was unstable. What was the reason for this decision? I had no idea other than the fact that it was public knowledge that I had a mental health history. The genuine concern I was having for my son now led me to be, once again, forcibly separated from him.

I had no idea where I was being taken since the officer drove in the complete opposite direction of where I requested to go. I continued to protest from the back seat of the police car. I was ignored. I believed that my life was to be ended as the officer sped recklessly into the night. At first, I did not recognize where we were when the car finally stopped. Then I saw the hospital sign. I felt some relief. I was still handcuffed as the police officer escorted me into the emergency room. Once again, I told him that I wanted to be admitted voluntarily. Instead of a response, he began writing on some type of form; a form that I knew would seal my fate, so I shouted as loud as I could, "I want to be voluntarily admitted." I spoke loud enough that everyone in the room heard me including the woman seated at the admission desk. The officer removed the handcuffs leaving me to stare at the blood on my wrist as he dropped the form on the desk of the receptionist and walked out the door.

I spent hours in the emergency room. The only "care" I received during that time was for me to provide a urine and blood sample. I never spoke to anyone who identified themselves as a doctor or mental health professional. I knew I would not test positive for drugs or alcohol, so I expected once I was evaluated I would be released. When I was told I was going to be transported to another facility, it became clear I was not being released. I did not recognize the name of the facility, nor was it clear to me why I was being taken there. Once I arrived at this facility, I learned it was a place where people are sent to for drug and alcohol detoxification. I was not alone in the confusion. The intake personnel, after reviewing my information, appeared perplexed asking each other, "Why is she here?" I sat there without any explanation myself. It was apparent they did not understand why I was brought there as I did not test positive for drugs or alcohol, plus I had medical insurance—it turns out the rehab facility primarily serves as a dumping ground for patients without insurance. I felt their remorse as they explained they had no option but to admit me anyway because of the official paperwork that had accompanied me.

If only Michael were home. His scheduled return was in just a couple days. If he were here, this would not be happening to me. He would have known how to handle the situation preventing it from ever getting to this point.

But it did happen. In fact, even worse things happened as a result of the proceeding events. While in the facility, I was dangerously overmedicated. No one listened to me nor did anyone seem to care, not even the doctor. I was assaulted by another patient and nearly committed to a state hospital. This was not a nightmare that I could wake up from. Rather it was the worst hospitalization I had ever experienced. Over the years, I had learned that a psychiatric patient still has rights. I was saved from a forced long and dangerous incarceration—without any formal charges or a trial of any kind—because of this knowledge. As soon as I could, I began to fight for my own freedom and sought for a way to obtain my release.

Before my release was finalized, Michael returned home from his trip. On the day of my scheduled release, the investigator from the Department of Children and Families contacted Michael. The investigator told him that if he did not sign a restraining order against me that our son would be removed from his custody as well. Michael felt as if his hand was forced to sign the order and that he had no other choice. I was released, but I had nowhere to go. I could not be with my son, nor could I be with my husband. Christmas, one of my favorite holidays, would soon be upon us--and my life would never be the same.

On the day I was accused of being an unfit mother and literally dragged out of my house, I was burdened by stress and sleep deprived, but I was clearly rational and in no way a danger to myself or anyone else. I had been receiving medical care and treatment for more than six years. I was not seeing visions or hearing voices. On the basis of what my 8-year-old son told his pediatrician, a man unqualified to make any kind of psychiatric evaluation, and on the authority of a DCF investigator who had no medical training whatsoever, my civil rights were trampled and my voice ignored. There was no professional, qualified evaluation of any kind before my forcible incarceration. Five years after this incident, I learned that our local sheriff's office began utilizing first responders who are trained in crisis intervention. This is a start, but more safeguards need to be in place to ensure that no one else has to endure what my family and I did.

To this day, I do not know what actually happened at my son's school. After this incident, I learned that as a result of 9/11, the schools in our area conducted "lock down" drills. At that time, I had no knowledge of these drills, but my understanding now is that a "lock down" occurs when there is a hijack situation at a school. I will always wonder if a drill was being conducted back during that time or if an actual situation was occurring. Maybe they assumed I knew something about the situation. To me, this seems to be the only explanation as to why the authorities would panic and treat me in the manner that they did.

As I write this, my family and I have been miraculously restored. I am happy and healthy, and Michael and I have a strong marriage. Our son is growing into the kind of young man who would make any parent proud. But we went through hell to get here, and almost all of it was entirely unnecessary.

It literally took years after the onset of postpartum psychosis before I was adequately diagnosed by a professional in the field of mental illness related to childbearing. Once I was able to receive the diagnosis, bipolar illness with a postpartum onset, I began the struggle to find and afford the appropriate care for my condition. Despite all of the difficulties and setbacks I encountered, I never for a single moment gave up the fight to be well. At the time of my commitment in 2003, although I still needed to find a new doctor, I was still seeing my therapist regularly; in fact, as soon as I began to experience stress while Michael was gone, I contacted her to request an earlier appointment and ask for assistance with a psychiatric referral. Although I was also still under the care of the endocrinologist I had begun to see after my possible miscarriage in New York City, I knew I would need to remain under the care of a psychiatrist as well.

Our finances were such, as a result of a change in our insurance plan, I was forced to leave my previous psychiatrist. When my therapist referred me to another psychiatrist, the earliest appointment I could obtain was in February. She was able to get this appointment moved up to January after I was forcibly hospitalized when my husband was away.

What happened to me in December cut across all the plans I had made and swept away all the research I had done up to that point. It is sobering to think that, at a stroke of a pen, one individual was able to start in motion, with really no evidence or personal accountability, a bureaucratic process in which I had no say and was forced to be my own advocate. Even an accused serial killer gets a defense attorney.

As a result of this process, my son was separated from me for months—despite the fact that I had never been accused, much less charged, with any form of abuse or neglect. How did this help an 8-year-old boy who had already been traumatized by the separation from his mom in the early part of his life? I will never understand how those involved thought their actions were in the best interest of my son and our family.

Everyone is different and every situation is unique. There is no one-size-fits-all solution to health care. In fact, I would say that the belief that health care can be narrowed to a specific drug or treatment for a specific set of symptoms is one of the biggest limitations of our current health care system. If you are dealing with any serious illness, you are going to need a well-informed, knowledgeable doctor, of course, but you will need much more than this. Your emotional and mental welfare are every bit as important as your physical welfare and need to be a part of your treatment plan.

In my case, for example, the right therapist was crucial, as was having a strong support system. I would not be alive today were it not for the love and support of family and friends. Traditional medicine may acknowledge the importance of support by providing assistance with referrals for support groups and counseling. However, you have to examine these options carefully when choosing the one that meets your individual needs.

Usually though, you will actually be on your own in seeking the spiritual care you need. I was fortunate that at the end of 2003, a man I encountered, referred me to a couple, both are pastors, who shared my beliefs and helped me find, through prayer and study, the kind of healing that comes from the inside out. Traditional medicine alone is not enough for me. I encourage you to consider your own needs carefully and seek out the spiritual healing you need. I did learn along my journey that the help I needed was out there. Unfortunately, rather than have others see to it that I find it, I discovered that I would have to look for it on my own.

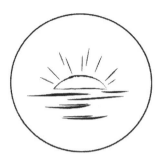

Chapter 15

Why This Story Must Be Told

My life is full of miracles. I have been blessed beyond anything I ever imagined. I have a wonderful, smart, happy, healthy, and well-adjusted, 17-year-old son. My marriage has survived storms that would surely cause many unions to sink. I have welcomed opportunities to assist families in need of support during their own difficulties related to the birth of a baby. I look back in amazement how I started out hoping I would be able to help at least one person. It's true that the challenges turned out to be greater than I could have imagined, but I tackled them the best I could.

I believe that we survive life's storms through the grace of God. Though the journey can be arduous, and though it may not be the voyage we expect it to be, or take us where we thought it should take us, grace is always available if we are willing to receive it. It's the willingness that takes courage, strength, and wisdom. We were never promised an easy road, but we were promised that we would never have to walk it alone.

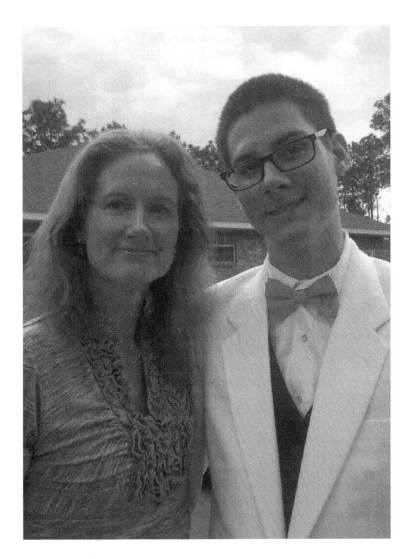

Me with my handsome son in 2013.

I am alive and well today because several things ultimately came together for me: I found the right doctors, medicines, therapist, and support. As a result of my struggle to find these things and recover from my illness, I have grown in both knowledge and wisdom. Good can come even from the toughest challenges we face and I am grateful for the gifts I have received, even those that have come at a high cost.

One of these gifts is a sense of purpose. I know what it is like to struggle to recover from an illness that is shrouded in ignorance and stigma. I know how hard the struggle can be to find the treatment and services you need in a medical system that often fails to honor the patient's voice in recovery. I know, intimately, how much these factors impact women and their families, and I am determined to be part of a solution that makes information about mental illness related to childbearing available to every woman and her family; insures that appropriate, professional treatment and counseling are accessible to the women and families that need them; and works to prevent these illnesses. No one should have to go through what my family and I did, but unfortunately many do.

I know what it is like to be among the lost, those who are tossed about in the stormy seas of a sudden, terrifying illness like postpartum psychosis. I know what it is like to fear that there is no safe harbor anywhere, and that you will be hurled against the rocks. I survived the storm, but many women still do not. Through PSI, and other organizations like it, I continue my efforts to be a lifeline for other women and families in this situation and to do what I can to help create a network of lifelines throughout the world. Together, we can make sure no one is lost in the storm.

Another gift I have received is learning that I am whole and healthy today because I learned to take as much care of my spiritual health, as I did my physical health. I believe that this is an essential part of recovery from not only mental illness related to childbearing, but all types of mental illness. Neglecting this aspect can make recovery much more difficult. However, this kind of care is intensely personal and specific to the needs of the individual's spirit.

Spiritual care generally lies outside the realm of traditional medicine, but it should be supported by non-judgmental medical professionals who respect one's spiritual needs. In my case, as often happens, too many of the medical professionals I saw simply wrote off my spiritual struggles as a physical symptom of my illness that needed to be suppressed or managed. But I found that I could not fully heal until I integrated spiritual healing into my treatment plan. I have since found that this is also true for many others, and the medical professionals who treat anyone experiencing mental illness should routinely acknowledge this factor.

As I recovered physically, mentally, emotionally, and spiritually, the next steps in my own journey began to unfold before me. I knew from bitter experience just how essential support is in overcoming mental illness related to childbearing—or any form of mental illness. In the early days of postpartum psychosis, the isolation I felt had been almost as difficult to bear as any of the symptoms. I longed to connect with someone who could understand what I was going through, and when I became stable myself, I wanted to make sure other women did not have to face one of the most difficult passages in their lives alone.

By early 2002, I had provided emotional and informational support to a number of women, but that spring I was blessed with an opportunity that would allow me to share my story to a much wider audience. It grew out of the Andrea Yates tragedy and the sensationalized, often inaccurate media coverage that surrounded it. A freelance writer, Liz Welch, hired by a national magazine to write a more positive, balanced story contacted Postpartum Support International, and Jane Honikman put her in touch with me.

I spoke with Liz and we hit it off immediately. I was excited to discover that the article she was writing would appear in *Glamour* magazine. It would reach millions of women and I could tell the story I thought the public needed to hear in the light of the Andrea Yates tragedy: Mental illness related to childbearing can strike women from all walks of life, but it is treatable and often preventable. Women do not have to suffer needlessly, and their stories do not have to end in tragedy. Liz was excited and thought she'd found the right person for the article. We were eager to start work as soon as possible.

But there was one hurdle to overcome. Shortly after we spoke, Liz called me back to say, "I know you're perfect for the story, but my editor isn't so sure. He wants someone

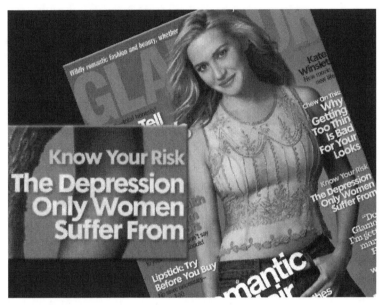

Cover of the February 2002 issue of Glamour Magazine with highlight of the article

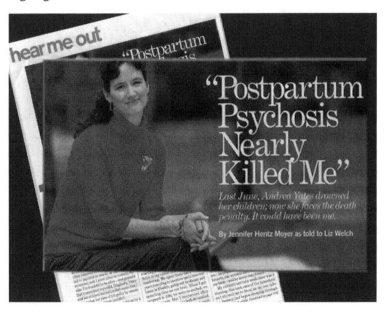

Photos of the February 2002 Glamour Magazine article

who can understand what Andrea Yates went through, but did not have psychosis herself."

Frustrating as it was, I almost had to laugh. The editor had demonstrated, in just one sentence, one of the reasons my story needed to be told—as other stories of so many women who have suffered postpartum psychosis—need to be told. Postpartum psychosis, or any other form of psychosis, for that matter, doesn't turn a woman into a monster, and it doesn't just happen to "crazy" people—i.e., the kind most people would rather avoid and never know. As for the editor wanting insight from someone "who hadn't had psychosis," I frankly thought that was ludicrous. Would he insist that only someone who'd never actually been there could write an article on China? As diplomatically as I could I asked, "How does he expect someone to understand if she has not had postpartum psychosis?"

Liz agreed and went to battle for me. He asked to see a picture of me. Apparently it took the picture to convince him. I guess he thought I looked like a "normal" person. I like to think that he became educated as I hoped the readers of the article would be. We are, in fact, "normal" people. Mental illness related to childbearing strikes sisters, daughters, coworkers, and friends.

Although the work Liz and I did on the article was time consuming and though it was, at times, difficult and painful to revisit many of my memories during the first year of my son's life, I am grateful for the experience. The freelance writer and the employees from *Glamour* Magazine who finalized the article treated me with complete respect and dignity. Even the photographers that came to my home for the photo shoot made me feel comfortable and that I should have no shame; ultimately, *Glamour* treated the then very controversial topic of postpartum psychosis with a high level of professionalism.

Most importantly of all, I learned that something positive came out of the article. Not long after the magazine became available in February 2002, it made an impact. I was told of one woman who read the article and showed up in a counselor's office with the magazine in her hand saying she knew she was in need of help after reading the article. Learning this was encouraging as I now knew the article was able to help at least one woman who was experiencing mental health challenges related to childbearing.

It was for that woman, and for all the women like her, that in March 2003, I agreed to appear on CNN's program, *The Point*. The producer that contacted me had read the article while in her doctor's waiting room. She wanted me to share some of the details of my own illness and give viewers my perspective on the Andrea Yates case. Though I was nervous, as it would be my first television appearance, and it was to be aired live, I knew it was necessary to speak openly about postpartum psychosis and share intimate details of my private life at such a far-reaching level. The stigma surrounding mental illnesses in general, and mental illnesses related to childbearing in particular, is difficult to overcome.

But it must be done as it is part of the story as well. What happened to me and to thousands of other women was not shameful and I thought of no reason to keep my experience silent.

It was time for the interview and I had no idea the specific questions that would be asked. So there was no way I could prepare, but when Anderson Cooper, the host, asked the controversial question, "Should Andrea Yates go to prison?" I did not hesitate to answer.

I confidently replied, "No, she should not. She needs proper medical treatment and she should be in a hospital, not a prison...I understand the living hell she and her family have been through." It was almost two years after the tragedy when I appeared on the program. The court trial was ongoing, so I was not surprised that this question was asked as it was being hotly debated. The tragedy had opened up a Pandora's Box, creating an intense and emotionally charged topic. That tragedy, as well as the many tragedies that do not make national attention, contributed to my reason for writing this book. Mental illnesses related to childbearing are treatable, and the majority of the anguish that Andrea Yates and her family went through was preventable.

For the most part, "going public" was a positive experience for me. A national platform allowed me to raise awareness about mental illnesses related to childbearing in a way I never could have done otherwise. I began to accept speaking engagements and additional interviews. Now, 12 years later, the public is much more aware of these illnesses.

Much of the awareness conveyed to the public comes from the media that either contributes to the stigma of mental illness or helps in educating and eliminating the stigma of mental illness. Unfortunately the media continues to create the stigma rather than help lessen it. Despite the misinformation, many of us work persistently and diligently to change the perception and understanding of mental illness. I am thankful that our relentless efforts are making a difference. Although we still have much further to go, treatment and support for mental illness related to childbearing has improved, and women now have many more options. I am glad to be one of those who participate in helping to make a difference.

But, not all of the response in going public with my story has been positive. I lost a few friends along the way. I guess they didn't understand mental illness is treatable and can be managed to the point of wellness. Some of those who learned more about my history were actually frightened of me. After I shared my story at my own church, for example, a woman came up to one of my friends and said, "You'd better watch out for that woman." People do not always let go of fear easily, and there is still a lot of ignorance and confusion about mental illness, in general. That is why I now do not pass up opportunities to talk about it. The more people I can talk with, the better the chances are that understanding can occur so that tragedies related to mental illness cease.

On Mother's Day in 2003, as I prepared to present my story to a large group of professionals, I wrote in my journal, "As I celebrate this Mother's Day, I can't help but think of the mothers who are not here because of the tragedy of mental illness related to childbearing. Help my voice be a representative of all those unable to speak out."

My own mother's sudden death in 2003 brought home to me in a whole new way how greatly mental illness related to childbearing can affect a family. My mother was part of my life for more than 36 years. She was a giving, caring, unselfish person who raised eight children in a loving home. She was my teacher, caregiver, best friend, and spiritual mentor; my life has been blessed in so many ways because she was a part of it. Her death was among the greatest sorrows I have ever experienced, but grief taught me how fortunate I had been. What would my life have been like, I asked myself, if she had not been there? What would my son's life be like now if I wasn't here?

Postpartum psychosis, in which a woman loses touch with reality after giving birth, is the rarest of the mental illnesses related to childbearing, but it is also the most serious. It was first recognized in 1850, and occurs after approximately 1.1-4 of deliveries.[1] The one thing most people do not know about postpartum psychosis is the risk of infanticide or suicide, is exceptionally low, and though media coverage often suggests otherwise, the risk of suicide is by far the greater of the two. The onset of postpartum psychosis is usually sudden, with symptoms that include delusions

---

1   Gaynes et. al. (2005). The estimate is approximate because there is still no diagnostic code for postpartum psychosis and cases are often mistaken for postpartum depression.

and/or hallucinations, feelings of extreme irritation, hyperactivity, and sleeplessness that can result in significant mood changes and impaired decision making ability.

Due to its severity and the risk to the mother and her baby, immediate treatment of postpartum psychosis is imperative. Unfortunately, it is estimated that fewer than 20 percent of women who suffer from symptoms ever talk to their health care providers about them. Mental illness in the United States is still stigmatized and women do not want their doctors, or anybody else, to think that they are "crazy," or that they are unfit mothers. Too often, postpartum psychosis can be misdiagnosed as postpartum depression, which is still a serious illness, but not as immediately threatening to the woman's health as postpartum psychosis can be. For both of these reasons, women do not receive the appropriate medical care, or receive it only after a great deal of suffering, as I did. This is a tragedy since women who receive properly targeted treatment usually respond very well, though I learned through my own experience that often it can be followed by depression before one completely recovers.

Every mother has a voice, but not every voice can be heard. The women who do not receive the treatment they need all too often become the silent, missing mothers. Those of us who lift our voices do so for those who no longer can.

I believe that each of us is a unique and beloved child of God. No one's life story is exactly like that of another. I can only tell you my story; every woman who suffers from mental illness related to childbearing has a story of her own. When we weave all of our stories together, each told in its own way by a woman speaking in her own voice, our families and communities grow in compassion, understanding, and wisdom. That is why every voice is important and another reason why I decided to write this book.

Ilylene Barsky once told me, "We are healed through helping others." Sharing my story has helped heal me in so many ways. It has especially helped in healing my spirit. When I was first struck with postpartum psychosis, it seemed to me that I had lost my voice completely. I wept, screamed in terror, and called for help; no one seemed to hear. I was treated like something broken or contaminated, so I became ashamed. I blamed myself for my illness, and the hardship and pain it caused all of my family.

As I began to heal, I found my own voice again and learned to make it heard. I came out of the darkness. The silence stopped and I spoke up in order to claim my right to be a partner in my own treatment and recovery. And I learned to put aside shame, guilt, and embarrassment. The onset of postpartum psychosis eight weeks after the birth of my son was a heartbreaking catastrophe, not a crime. I did not deserve the forcefulness, intimidation, imprisonment, neglect, and abuse that I encountered during the years I struggled to regain my health. No woman does.

When I speak to others, whether individually or to a larger audience, I often compare my experience to that of a woman who has been raped. It's a harsh and shocking comparison, and that's deliberate. I want it to make people think about the way our society treats those who have been stigmatized. The harshness of the word "rape" strips away all of the euphemisms we use to distance ourselves from stark realities. But the comparison is apt as well; both experiences are forced, violent, and abusive. Both violate and reduce women to helpless victims and steal their autonomy.

I believe that much of the abuse and neglect that women with postpartum psychosis and other mental illnesses related to childbearing experience springs from the public's fear and ignorance. Every so often, as in the Andrea Yates case, there's another sensationalized, tragic story about a woman who has harmed or killed her own children. The news circulates and the media dwells on the horror which fuels public outrage. Then the story will die down, and we'll hear no more about mental illness related to childbearing until the next tragedy occurs. We won't hear about the women who take their own lives in despair, or those who suffer the terrifying pain of postpartum psychosis without access to proper care, or even the stories of women who win their own battles against fear and ignorance and manage to heal. This is what groups like Postpartum Support International are committed to changing. Many are working to change the narrative from sensation to education and from judgment to understanding.

The desperate women who injure or kill their own children don't do so because they are evil. They do so because they are ill; so frightened and so detached from reality that they can no longer make reasonable decisions. How does it help anyone to punish them? Why not concentrate on changing the health care system that often fails them? Why not concentrate on ensuring that health care professionals are properly equipped and trained to diagnose and treat mental illness related to childbearing? Why not make sure that training includes the most up-do-date knowledge and treatments available? Why does every community not have a resource network to refer women and families? Though in actuality a postpartum-onset mental illness can occur for up to two years following the birth of a child, here in the USA many medical textbooks, and nearly all insurance companies, still define the "postpartum period" as lasting only four to six weeks. Why is there still, more than 160 years after it was first recognized, no diagnostic code for postpartum psychosis? Under the current definition of the postpartum period, it is hard for women to obtain proper treatment, and without a specific diagnostic code, how can there be accurate data or research on postpartum psychosis?

Finally, why don't we ensure that all women and their families have access to accurate information about mental illness related to childbearing and to timely, professional care? Perhaps the greatest tragedy in this litany of troubles is that these illnesses are not only curable, they are also largely preventable.

Other industrialized countries do a much better job of treating mental illness related to childbearing. It's difficult to understand why the United States continues to fall behind in this area given our historic record of achieving all we have as a nation; it is difficult to escape the conclusion that we appear to choose not to make a commitment to doing a better job treating any type of mental illness. Why not change that?

My illness came on suddenly, and it was severe. It would take me a very long time to understand what had happened to me, and to begin to heal. Today, I am convinced that the suffering I went through was needlessly prolonged because I did not receive appropriate care from the beginning. Despite a series of hospitalizations, and despite years of consultations with psychiatrists, doctors, therapists, and counselors, I had to wait more than six years before I was able to see a doctor who specialized in mental illness related to childbearing. It was as a result of his diagnosis in 2003 that I finally began to bring the puzzle pieces together

One critical piece of the puzzle was given to me in early 2004 by the psychiatrist I was able to see after I was horrifically taken from my son at the end of 2003 while Michael was out of the country. This psychiatrist was able to share with me an article from a psychiatric journal published less than two months before my first visit with him—the timing almost seemed ironic to me. It addressed the relationship between postpartum psychosis and bipolar disorder. The article included clinical information, but I understood the substance of the article. What I learned was that a woman who suffers from postpartum psychosis should routinely be put on mood stabilizing medication, regardless of whether or not she has a previous history of bipolar illness. If she is instead placed on an antidepressant, which often happens since postpartum psychosis is often misdiagnosed as post-partum depression, she typically experiences many more up and down cycles in her recovery. I cried when I read the article; in a few pages it encapsulated years of my own history.

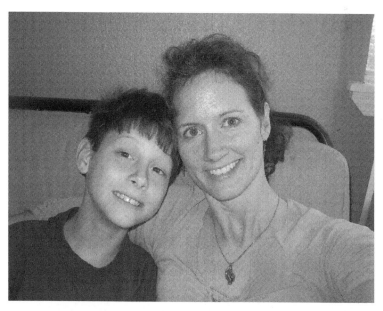

My son and I in November 2004, over 16 months since my mom's death and the diagnosis of bipolar disorder, postpartum onset.

For me, the article was life changing; it made sense of all the times I'd struggled to put my life back together, only to fail again just when it seemed things were going well. It explained why it had been so hard for me to handle the normal stresses of day-to-day life I'd managed so easily before. I had always been a healthy, competent woman who rarely needed an aspirin, much less a medicine cabinet full of prescription drugs. Why had I been unable to become that woman once again? I think the article helped me lay aside the last, lingering echoes of guilt that this was all somehow my fault.

But I began to ponder the questions, "Why did it take years before I heard any of this?" and "Why was I not given a mood stabilizer immediately after postpartum psychosis struck me?" The article itself may have been "cutting edge," but it referenced material and research that had been available for decades. The more I thought about that, the angrier I became and, yes, that is another reason I wrote this book. There is nothing wrong with a little righteous anger, if it is properly directed. I decided to take mine and put it to good use.

Or at least I did, for a while. The truth is that even justifiable anger can take you only so far. Over time, I found that it wears you down. I let mine cool and found that I could replace it with compassion and understanding. I knew I still had a lot to learn about the condition that is now my companion for the rest of my life. So, I made "friends" with bipolar disorder. I got to know it and let it teach me what

I will need to do to stay healthy as long as we're living to-gether. Having the compassion and understanding that my "friend" helped me gain, I now help others to be hopeful that they too can become "friends" when they are faced with the "enemy" of mental illness.

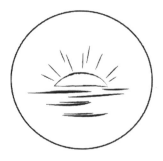

Afterword

Despite the diagnosis of bipolar disorder, postpartum onset being placed upon me more than ten years ago, no longer is it the controller of my life. Thankfully, I've been stable for more than seven years now. During that time, I've learned how to better manage my health through a combination of good nutrition, regular exercise, the right medication, appropriate therapy, and a strong support system. I would not be alive today without these things, and I am grateful for the caring professionals who have treated me with dignity and respect, and helped me to heal. It took a heartbreaking struggle to find them, one that I would not wish on any woman, but that does not diminish the good deed that each one of them carried out, which ultimately helped me reach this point in my life.

Today I continue treatment for bipolar disorder. I had a setback in January 2005, when the anti-psychotic medication I was taking at that time, began to affect my blood sugar. After all I had been through I believed I had no option but to continue taking it. However, my doctor did lower the dosage. I began to take on more responsibilities, not yet having all the tools I would need to move forward in my life. I now know that I was ill equipped to recognize and understand the symptoms of bipolar disorder. One must understand what to expect or what to look for if one is to prepare and address a potential outcome. With the lack of knowledge and tools that were necessary, coupled with the lower dosage in my medication, I once again found myself hospitalized in January 2005.

This hospitalization was different. Despite the fact that it put my marriage on the path of destruction, it in time became a blessing. I was put on a medicine that the hospital doctor had watched for a year before prescribing it to her own patients. She explained the benefits she was seeing. We even shared opinions regarding the limitations of providing treatment under a health care system that is primarily profit-driven.

In taking the new medication, I had to be weaned off the old medication. During this process, I began to have flu-like symptoms along with general aches and pains. I knew I was not sick with the flu, so this caused me alarm. I had been discharged from the hospital by this point, so I thought to call the endocrinologist thinking that it could be related to changes in my blood sugar. He was able to explain to me, that although it was not his area of expertise, his understanding is that often the body goes through an adjustment period during medication changes. He went on to say that these symptoms typically pass in a period of time. I felt a sense of relief as he told me this as I had considered stopping the medication. This would not have been a good choice.

After I was completely off the old medication and solely on the new one, not only did the symptoms subside, but the medication began to help me with other symptoms which, through a support group, I learned were symptoms related to bipolar disorder. The symptoms I learned about but did not recognize prior to attending the support group were: I could be unreasonable, argumentative, have excessive energy which interfered with my sleep, and I believed I could accomplish anything despite my limitations. I thought how ironic it was that I received this information from individuals that were not even mental health professionals.

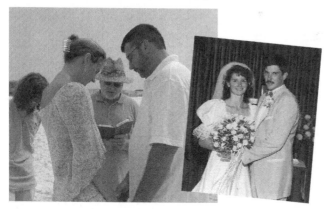

Wedding day for Michael and I in July 1988. Pastor John blessing Michael and I in July 2008 on our vow renewal day in celebration of our 20 years of marriage.

My love and deep gratitude goes to my husband Michael, who traveled with me down a very tough road. The darkness seemed to overtake our marriage to the point that it would not survive, but it did. Our commitment to each other to stay on the road, when so many others do not, remains today. It took courage to travel this road. In the summer of 2013, we celebrated our 25th wedding anniversary. We look forward to at least another 25 years together. Our son has turned into an amazing, talented, and compassionate young man as he prepares to graduate from high school. The future of our family now shines bright.

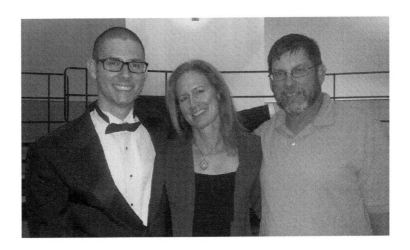

References

Ackerman, S. (2011). *Supermom: A postpartum anxiety survival story.* Burlington, IN: iUniverse.

Armstrong, H. (2009). *It sucked and then I cried: How I had a baby, a breakdown, and a much needed margarita.* New York: Gallery Books.

Barnes, D. L., & Balber, L. (2007). *The journey to parenthood: Myths, reality and what really matters.* London: Radcliffe Publishing.

Beck, C. T., & Driscoll, J. W. (2005). *Postpartum mood and anxiety disorders: A guide.* Burlington, MA: Jones and Bartlett.

Bennett, S. (2007). *Postpartum depression for dummies.* Hobeken, NJ: Wiley Publishing.

Bennett, S. (2008). *Pregnant on Prozac: The essential guide to making the best decision for you and your baby.* Guilford, CT: The Globe Pequot Press.

Bennett, S., & Indman, P. (2010). *Beyond the blues: Understanding and treating prenatal and postpartum depression and anxiety.* San Jose, CA: Moodswing Press.

Blumfield, W. (1992). *Life after birth: Every woman's guide to the first year of motherhood.* Rockport, MA: Element Books Ltd.

Carp, H. (2003). *The happiest baby on the block: The new way to calm crying and help your newborn baby sleep longer.* New York: Random House.

Chaudron, L., & Pies, R.W. (2003). The relationship between postpartum psychosis and bipolar disorder: A review. *Journal of Clinical Psychiatry, 64*(11), 1284-1292.

Cohen, L. S., & Nonacs, R. (2005). *Mood and anxiety disorders during pregnancy and postpartum (review of psychiatry).* Arlington, VA: American Psychiatric Publishing.

Cozad, S., & Cozad, C. *Mama's voyage.* Retrieved from http://www.mamasvoyage.com/book.htm

Dalfen, A. (2009). *When baby brings the blues: Solutions for postpartum depression.* Chichester, West Sussex, England: John Wiley and Sons.

Dix, C. (1988). *The new mother syndrome: Coping with postpartum stress and depression.* New York: Pocket Books.

Dowling, C. (1993). *You mean I don't have to feel this way? New help for depression, anxiety, and addiction.* New York: Bantam Books.

Dunnewold, A. (2007). *Even June Cleaver would forget the juice box: Cut yourself some slack and (still raise great kids) in the age of extreme parenting.* Deerfield Beach, FL: Health Communications, Inc.

Dunnewold, A., & Sanford, D. G. (1994). *Postpartum survival guide.* Oakland, CA: New Harbinger Publications.

Feingold, S. B. (2013). *Happy endings, new beginnings: Navigating postpartum disorders.* Far Hills, NJ: New Horizon Press.

Ferber, M.D., & Jane, S., (1997). *A woman doctor's guide to depression.* New York: Hyperion.

Finkelstein, B. (2009). *Delivery from darkness: A Jewish guide to prevention and treatment of postpartum depression.* Hanuet, NY: Philipp Feldheim.

Fran, R. (1994). *What happened to mommy?* Eastman, GA: R.D. Eastman Publishing.

Georgiopoulos, A., Bryan, T.L., Wollan, B., & Yawn, B.P. (2001). Routine screening for postpartum depression. *Journal of Family Practice, 50*(2), 117-122.

Gyoerkoe, K. L., & Wiegartz, P. (2009). *The pregnancy and postpartum anxiety workbook: Practical skills to help you overcome anxiety, worry, panic attacks, obsessions, and compulsions.* Oakland, CA: New Harbinger Publications.

Halvorson, S.C. (2004). *Beth: A story of postpartum psychosis.* Bloomington, IN: 1st Books (Author House).

Hamilton, J. A., & Harberger, P.N. (1992). *Postpartum psychiatric illness: A picture puzzle.* Philadelphia: University of Pennsylvania Press.

Hart, A. D. (1993). *Dark clouds, silver linings.* Colorado Springs, CO: Focus on the Family Publishing.

Honikman, J.I. (2002). *I'm listening.* Santa Barbara, CA: Studio E Books.

Isnardi, W. (2011). *Nobody told me: My battle with postpartum depression and obsessive-compulsive disorder.* Long Island, NY: Legwork Team Publishing.

Kendall-Tackett, K. A. (2009). *Depression in new mothers: Causes, consequences, and treatment alternatives, 2nd Edition.* London: Routledge.

Kleiman, K. R. (2001). *The postpartum husband: Practical solutions for living with postpartum depression.* Bloomington, IN: Xlibris.

Kleiman, K. (2005). *What am I thinking? Having a baby after postpartum depression.* Bloomington, IN: Xlibris Corporation.

Kleiman, K., & Raskin, V.D. (1994). *This isn't what I expected: Overcoming postpartum depression.* New York: Bantam Books.

Kleiman, K., & Wenzel, A. (2010). *Dropping the baby and other scary thoughts: Breaking the cycle of unwanted thoughts in motherhood*. New York: Routledge.

Lasalandra, S. M. (2005). *A daughter's touch: A journey of a mother trying to come to terms with postpartum depression*. Franklin Lakes, NJ: Quattro M Publishing.

Madsen, L. (1994). *Rebounding from childbirth: Toward emotional recovery*. Westport, CT: Bergin and Garvey.

Maley, B. (2002). Creating a postpartum depression support group, *AWHONN Lifelines, February/March*, 62-65.

Martini, A. (2008). *Hillbilly gothic: A memoir of madness and motherhood*. New York: Atria Books.

McRoberts, S. (2007). *The lifter of my head: How God sustained me during postpartum depression*. Mustang, OR: Tate Publishing.

McGee, R. S. (1985). *The search for significance*. Houston, TX: Rapha Publishing.

Milgrom, J., Martin, P. R., & Negri, L. M. (2000). *Treating postnatal depression: A psychological approach for health care practitioners*. Chicester, West Sussex, England: John Wiley and Sons.

Miller, L. (1999). *Postpartum mood disorders (clinical practice)*. Arlington, VA: American Psychiatric Publishing.

Moyer, J. H., & Welch, L. (2002). Postpartum psychosis nearly killed me, *Glamour, February*.

Peck, M. S. (1993). *Further along the road less traveled*. New York: Touchstone.

Placksin, S. (2000). *Mothering the new mother*. New York: Newmarket Press.

Resnick, S. K. (2000). *Sleepless days*. New York: St. Martin's Press.

Rosenberg, R., Greening, J., & Windell, D. (2003). *Conquering postpartum depression*. Darby, PA: Diane Pub Co.

Sabraw, S., Levy, M., & Sanders, D. (2002). Moms who kill. *Psychology Today, December*.

Shields, B. (2005). *Down came the rain: My journey through postpartum depression*. New York: Hyperion.

Vermont Postpartum Task Force. (2002). *Life after childbirth*. Retrieved from: http://www.vermontpostpartumtaskforce.org/

Wood, L.C., Cooper, D.S., & Ridgeway, E.C. (1995). *Your thyroid: A home reference*. New York: Ballantine Books.

Resources

If you are afraid or planning to harm yourself, your baby, or others, you need to call your health care provider, dial 911 (emergency services), or go to the nearest hospital emergency room. If you are in crisis, someone is available to talk with you now. Please know you are not alone in this. An understanding person is waiting to hear from you and help you.

The information listed here is not intended to diagnose or treat any medical or psychological condition. Please consult with your health care provider for individual advice regarding your own situation.

Emergency and Mental Health Related
National Suicide Prevention Lifeline
1-800-273-8255
1-800-273-TALK
www.suicidepreventionlifeline.org

American Association of Suicidology
AAS is a membership organization for all those involved in suicide prevention and intervention, or touched by suicide. AAS is a leader in the advancement of scientific and programmatic efforts in suicide prevention through research, education and training, the development of standards and resources, and survivor support services.
www.suicidology.org/web/guest/home

Baby Safe Haven: Do Not Abandon Your Newborn/ AMT Children of Hope Safe Haven Program

If you are pregnant and afraid to tell anyone, or if you do not know what to do with your newborn baby, call for help or take your baby to any hospital emergency room. Your secret and baby will be safe. The police will not be called. You will not have to answer any questions. Confidential help and support are available to you

1-877-796-HOPE
1-877-796-4673
www.amtchildrenofhope.com

Bring Change 2 Mind

Working together to erase the stigma of mental illness, Bring Change 2 Mind is a national anti-stigma campaign founded by Glenn Close, The Balanced Mind Foundation, Fountain House, and Garen and Shari Staglin of the International Mental Health Research Organization (IMHRO), aimed at removing misconceptions about mental illness. The idea was born out of a partnership between Glenn Close and Fountain House, where Glenn volunteered in order to learn more about mental illness, which both her sister, Jessie Close, and nephew, Calen Pick, live with.

www.bringchange2mind.org

Child Abuse Prevention

Childhelp USA National Child Abuse Hotline
1-800-422-2253
1-800-4-A-CHILD
www.childhelpusa.org

Citizens Commission on Human Rights

The Citizens Commission on Human Rights (CCHR) is a nonprofit mental health watchdog, responsible for helping to enact more than 150 laws protecting individuals from abusive or coercive practices.

www.cchr.org

Depression and Bipolar Support Alliance
DBSA offers information on depression and bipolar disorder as well as listings to patient support groups across the USA.
www.dbsalliance.org

HRSA/US Department of Health and Human Services Site on Perinatal Depression
Download or order free booklet, *Depression During and After Pregnancy: A Resource for Women, Their Families and Friends* (English and Spanish).
www.mchb.hrsa.gov / pregnancyandbeyond / depression /

Marce Society International
The Marcé Society is an international society for the understanding, prevention and treatment of mental illness related to childbearing. The principal aim of the society is to promote, facilitate, and communicate about research into all aspects of the mental health of women, their infants, and partners around the time of childbirth.
www.marcesociety.com

MedEdPPD
Provides education and resources about perinatal mood disorders for professionals and the public in English and Spanish. Online curriculum available. Provides online video examples of the Baby Blues, Postpartum Depression, and Postpartum Psychosis.
www.MedEdPPD.org

Mental Health America
Mental Health America is dedicated to promoting mental health, preventing mental illness and substance use conditions, and achieving victory over mental illnesses and addictions through advocacy, education, research, and service.
www.nmha.org

Mental Health Counselors
Clinical mental health counselors provide flexible, consumer-oriented therapy that combines traditional psychotherapy with a practical, problem-solving approach to create a dynamic and efficient path for change and problem resolution. Here a few links to help you locate one in your area.
www.amhca.org/public_resources/default.aspx
www.1-800-therapist.com
therapists.psychologytoday.com/rms

NAMI: National Alliance on Mental Illness–Mental Health Support
The nation's largest nonprofit, grassroots mental health education, advocacy, and support organization.
www.nami.org

National Hopeline Network
1-800 SUICIDE
www.hopeline.com

The National Institute of Mental Health (NIMH)
The largest scientific organization in the world dedicated to research focused on the understanding, treatment, and prevention of mental illnesses.
www.nimh.nih.gov

National Suicide Prevention Lifeline
1-800-273-8255
1-800-273-TALK
www.suicidepreventionlifeline.org

Postpartum Depression Support Organizations in the US, Canada, UK, South Africa, Australia, and New Zealand
www.postpartumprogress.com/postpartum-depression-support-organizations-in-the-us-canada-uk-south-africa-australia-new-Zealand
Postpartum Depression Awareness CANADA

Postpartum Support International (PSI)
The non-profit organization providing resources with extensive social support network throughout the United States and worldwide. Multi-lingual information for health care providers and the public. Free weekly educational telephone group sessions, online support, and support for dads and military families also available.
www.postpartum.net

U.S. Food and Drug Administration
The Food and Drug Administration (FDA) is an agency within the U.S. Department of Health and Human Services. Protecting the public health by assuring that foods are safe, wholesome, sanitary, and properly labeled. They also monitor human and veterinary drugs, and vaccines and other biological products, and medical devices intended for human use to ensure that they are safe and effective.
www.medicinenet.com
Website for information on medications

Online Postpartum Depression Support Resources

www.postpartumdepression.yuku.com
www.ppdsupportpage.com
www.postpartumprogress.com
www.jennyslight.org
www.postpartummen.com
www.MedEdPPD.org

Resources Specific to Postpartum Psychosis

APP: Action Postpartum Psychosis
APP is a network of women across the UK and further afield who have experienced postpartum psychosis (PP). It is a collaborative project run by women who have experienced PP and academic experts from Birmingham and Cardiff Universities.
www.app-network.org

Healthy Mom, Happy Family: Understanding Pregnancy and Postpartum Mood and Anxiety Disorders
Preview a 13-minute video produced by Postpartum Support International. Available through www.postpartum.net, it helps reassure and educate new mothers, families, and helpers. The poignant stories in the video are complemented by up-to-date information from three experts in the field.

Personal Stories of Postpartum Psychosis
News report from BBC
http://www.bbc.com/news/health-19351270

The Symptoms of Postpartum Psychosis
A short video describing the symptoms of postpartum psychosis from Life Videopedia
http://on.aol.com/video/the-symptoms-of-postpartum-psychosis-512601313

Understanding Postpartum Psychosis by Teresa Twomey
Offering an understanding of postpartum psychosis, this riveting book explains what happens and why during this temporary and dangerous disorder that develops for some women rapidly after childbirth.
http://www.amazon.com/Understanding-Postpartum-Psychosis-Temporary-Madness/dp/0313353468/ref=sr_1_sc_1?s=books&ie=UTF8&qid=1328374500&sr=1-1-spell

Postpartum Psychosis: More than the Baby Blues
An article in H News, Canada's health care newspaper
http://hospitalnews.com/postpartum-psychosis-more-
than-the-baby-blues/

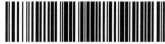
41140258R00150

Made in the USA
Charleston, SC
24 April 2015